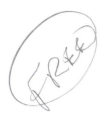
The Sexual Health of Men

The Sexual Health of Men

Edited by

Laura Serrant-Green

PhD MA BA RGN PGCE
Principal Development Fellow
School of Health
University of Wolverhampton

and

John McLuskey

MPH BSc RGN FETC
Associate Professor
School of Nursing
University of Nottingham

Foreword by

Alan White

Professor of Men's Health
Director, Centre for Men's Health
Leeds Metropolitan University

Radcliffe Publishing
Oxford • New York

Radcliffe Publishing Ltd
18 Marcham Road
Abingdon
Oxon OX14 1AA
United Kingdom

www.radcliffe-oxford.com
Electronic catalogue and worldwide online ordering facility.

British Library Cataloguing in Publication Data

A catalogue record for this book is available from the British Library.

ISBN-13: 978 1 84619 034 6

Typeset by 4Word Ltd, Bristol
Printed and bound by TJI Digital, Padstow, Cornwall

Contents

Foreword   vi
About the editors   viii
About the contributors   ix

1   Introduction   1
     Laura Serrant-Green and John McLuskey

2   Recasting masculinity: mapping out challenges and opportunities for
     public health   13
     Graham Holroyd, Denise Richardson and James Webb

3   Men and sexual health   27
     Laura Serrant-Green

4   Physical sexual ill health   37
     John McLuskey and Laura Serrant-Green

5   Psychosexual aspects of men's health   57
     Joy Hall

6   Sexual behaviour   83
     John McLuskey

7   Sexual health promotion for black and minority ethnic men   93
     Vanessa McFarlane and Laura Serrant-Green

8   Providing sexual health services for men   115
     Kevin Miles

Index   141

Foreword

In 2000 Yvette Cooper, the then Public Health Minister, launched a campaign aimed at young men in an attempt to reduce the number of teenage pregnancies under the strapline that boys were 'half the problem and half the solution'. What was relevant about this campaign is that it was the first real attempt by Government to acknowledge that men were equally responsible for the numbers of teenage pregnancies!

Up to that time all policy, and indeed all services, were almost entirely focused exclusively on women. Men were seen as feckless and apart from the push to get gay men to wear condoms and have safe sex as part of the reaction to the horrors of AIDs in the 1980s there were no real attempts to influence men's beliefs or behaviour around their sexual health. Sexual Education in schools for boys was rudimentary and tackled from a purely biological perspective; when girls were given their talk on puberty boys were sent out to play. Within the health services men didn't fair much better as there was not a lot of interest or attention paid to their sexual health. Prostate cancer was certainly not as prevalent as it is today, but there was scant research on either its cause or the best form of treatment, with castration being one of the main forms of treatment. Erectile dysfunction (ED), or to give its more value-laden term 'impotence' as was used, was seen purely as a psychological problem.

Men's 'sexual health' was therefore a side issue, one relegated to a brief mention in a medical or nursing textbook or to the top shelves of newsagent journals. Times have changed and as this book attests our awareness of the importance of men having good sexual health as both an intrinsic human right and also as a precursor to a more healthy society has certainly changed.

The call for greater work with boys in schools has never been more important, and this needs to start early to prepare boys for the challenges of adolescence and to give them the understanding both around sex and sexual health and also the confidence and knowledge to use health services appropriately. This must be seen as a priority as the UK still holds the dubious honour of having the highest rate of teenage pregnancy in Europe and among the highest incidence of sexually transmitted infections.

Erectile dysfunction is increasingly seen as a physical problem and indeed a 'sentinel' alarm for cardiovascular disorders with increasingly strong links to the metabolic syndrome. Until we get men generally, and health practitioners particularly, to recognise that a proper medical examination is the first stage for a man with ED, we run the risk of men turning towards dangerous alternatives. This is certainly seen with regard to the Internet, where recent estimates suggest that nearly 750,000 men buy drugs online, with a growing number of these drugs identified as counterfeit. In part this is due to men's anxieties about speaking to health professionals about sexual health problems but it is not helped by the continued constraints placed on the prescription of ED drugs, limiting legitimate treatment options for health professionals and making some men feel that it is futile to seek appropriate help.

The new Gender Equality Duty, which came into force with the 2006 Equality Act in April 2007, means that there is now a legal responsibility to ensure all health and social care policies meet the needs of both men and women. This book, with its detailed appraisal of what sexual health means to men, will be of great worth to those now trying to devise sexual health policy and local strategies that will ensure men are fully taken into consideration. It will also be of importance to those commissioned to purchase sexual healthcare services and to both practitioners and teachers who are tasked with both educating boys and men about their sexual health and with their treatment. In addition, this book will be of immense value to academics who are working in the field of men's health, gender studies, sociology, psychology and others in health or social care.

This authoritative book has set a new benchmark that others will be judged against.

Professor Alan White
Professor of Men's Health
Director, Centre for Men's Health
Leeds Metropolitan University

January 2008

About the editors

Laura Serrant-Green is Principal Development Fellow at the University of Wolverhampton. She is also a freelance researcher, trainer and educational consultant. She has previously been awarded the Mary Seacole Nursing Leadership Award, Smith and Nephew Research Fellowship and Florence Nightingale Travel Fellowship for her research work around black men and sexual health behaviour. She is currently editor of *Nurse Researcher*, an international journal of nursing and healthcare research methodology.

John McLuskey is an Associate Professor within the School of Nursing at the University of Nottingham. One of his key roles within the University is to lead a sexual health pathway. He is also a Director of the European Men's Health Development Foundation and has been Chair to the Foundation since 2005. This book has allowed him to join together his two areas of academic interest: sexual health and the health of men.

About the contributors

Joy Hall MSc, BEd, RN, DipNurs, RNT, BASRT, Accredited & UKCP Registered Psychosexual & Relationship Psychotherapist
Head of Division Women's Health, Birmingham City University
Since gaining her RN at Addenbrooke's Hospital in 1982, Joy has worked extensively in adult and sexual health nursing, and nurse education. Her particular area of interest is psychosexual health, and she became a qualified psychosexual and relationship therapist in 1997. She was formerly a member of the RCN Sexual Health Forum Committee and committee member for various groups with the British Association of Sexual & Relationship Therapists (BASRT).

Graham Holroyd MSc, BA, DipASCE, MIHE
Senior Lecturer, Lancashire School of Health and Postgraduate Medicine, University of Central Lancashire
Graham has a number of publications in the area of men and health. His current research interests include men and health, social capital and capacity building, social inclusion and community regeneration, applied to public health. He is a Co-director and past Chair of the European Men's Health Development Foundation.

Vanessa McFarlane BA
Health Promotion Specialist, Black and Asian Sexual Health, Nottingham City PCT
Vanessa has worked extensively in community and primary care-based services around health promotion, focussing on the needs of black and minority ethnic communities. She has a wealth of experience in community engagement and action research-focussed initiatives.

Kevin Miles PhD, MSc, DipTropNurs, DipNurs, RGN
Nurse Consultant in Sexual Health and HIV, Camden PCT
Honorary Lecturer, Centre for Sexual Health & HIV Research, University College London
Kevin's clinical work has predominately specialised in male sexual health, including targeted prevention and treatment services for men who have sex with men, male sex workers, homeless youth, adolescents and HIV-positive men. He completed an MSc in Sexually Transmitted Diseases in 1998 and his PhD (2002) focused on the evaluation of nurse-led sexual health services.

Denise Richardson MA, BSc
Senior Lecturer, Lancashire School of Health and Postgraduate Medicine,
University of Central Lancashire
Denise is a senior lecturer in the Lancashire School of Health and Postgraduate
Medicine, in the Faculty of Health at the University of Central Lancashire. She is
currently researching 'Women and the settlement of Irish tinsmith/traveller families
in Ireland since the 19th century: continuity and change' for her DPhil thesis at the
School of History and International Affairs, University of Ulster.

James Webb BSc
Postgraduate Student, Lancashire School of Health and Postgraduate Medicine,
University of Central Lancashire
James graduated from the University of Central Lancashire having achieved an MA
in Health Promotion and now works for a health communications agency in
London.

This book is dedicated to:

Robert McLuskey, my father, a man who understood the importance of sexual health as a father of nine.
John McLuskey

Graham, Robert, Jack and Helena, my family, who put up with discussions of men's sexual health far beyond the call of duty.
Laura Serrant-Green

CHAPTER 1

Introduction

Laura Serrant-Green and John McLuskey

This book will explore the challenges, constraints and opportunities for addressing and promoting the sexual health of men in Britain. It begins by considering many issues, including some of the ways in which sexual health has been defined in society, and discusses how the sexual health of men compared with that of women has received little attention from health researchers, policy makers and health service providers. It continues through the ensuing chapters to explore, highlight and critique some of the consequences of this for sexual health policy, service provision and healthcare practice. Ultimately the aims of the book are:

- To critically examine men's sexual health within personal, social and political contexts
- To provide a platform for reviewing the importance of integrating psychosocial and physical aspects into men's sexual healthcare provision
- To bring together expert evidence from the fields of sexual health research, education and practice

The book is aimed at health and social care professionals, e.g. nurses, social workers, health advisers, medics, sexual health service providers and others concerned about the sexual health and well-being of men. The authors hope that the book will provide a useful resource and add to the information available that focuses on the sexual health of men.

SEXUAL HEALTH AND BRITISH SOCIETY

The past few decades have seen increasing interest in sexual health as an area of concern for healthcare professionals and service providers in Britain. This has occurred against a backdrop of wider changes in healthcare policy, where the focus is primarily on prevention of ill health and promotion of healthy lifestyles.[1,2] Since the emergence of HIV and AIDS in the twentieth century, issues such as sexual health and the need to provide for what were previously viewed as private issues between individuals have entered the public sphere.[3–5] Sexual health is in general no longer simply a matter of a physical act with consequences for an individual, but is recognised by the Government, health and social care providers as an area of health need requiring planning, assessing and services to support it.[6,7]

However, the apparent recognition of a need to address sexual health issues at an individual and strategic level is juxtaposed by the silences that have developed around sexual health as a subject in itself and the way it has been addressed within a healthcare context. Discussions of sexual health as an area of need in health policy and the healthcare strategies used to promote it have been built around a very narrow view of what constitutes sexual health. This view had at its core an implicit assumption that the nature of sexual health was primarily concerned with physiological functioning.[8] In this context a tradition of sexual-health work has developed in healthcare practice where it is more likely to be associated with reproductive function, the investigation and treatment of sexually transmitted infections and the prevention of unplanned pregnancy.[9–11] As a result there exists in Britain a historical legacy of relatively little discussion amongst professionals, policy makers and service providers about any possible variation in people's understanding of sexual health and the consequences of this for diverse populations. This has occurred despite the fact that as far back as 1975 the World Health Organization (WHO) urged healthcare professionals to widen their views on sexual health away from pure epidemiology and sexual intercourse towards a more positive and holistic approach. They called for:

> The integration of the somatic, emotional, intellectual and social aspects of sexual being in ways that are positively enriching and that enhance personality, communication and love.[12]

In contrast to the situation in healthcare practice, the social sciences, particularly areas such as gender and cultural studies, have produced a vast array of literature investigating and discussing a wide variety of issues relating to sexual health, including sexuality, self-identity and social stigma. Of the studies investigating sexual health from a healthcare perspective, few have incorporated a person-centred approach. Up until the 1980s at least most continued with the push to 'measure' sexual health in terms of infection and pregnancy. In this environment little consideration was given to the wider components of sexual health and the possibility of variation in the associated sexual decision-making of different groups in society.[13] As a consequence, with the exception of HIV/AIDS, which will be commented on later, discussing 'sexual health' is to a great extent actually synonymous with 'sexual ill health' and disease, with epidemiological studies forming the main and often only source of research data.

The majority of the research conducted under this restricted interpretation of sexual health centred on medical treatments for specific diseases such as sexually transmitted infections (STIs), or took the form of large surveys conducted by public health departments. The contribution of person-centred or sociological approaches from healthcare professionals to this challenging area of health were conspicuous by their absence. The reasons for the lack of information or investigation into the nature and consequences of sexual health from a healthcare perspective are complex. Some of the possible influencing factors relate to wider social attitudes to sexual health as an issue in itself, while others are specifically associated with the response of healthcare providers to sexual health as an area of healthcare.

Research into sexual health is impeded by a variety of issues related to the nature of sex and sexual expression in society.[8] Sexual health has throughout history been inextricably associated with social taboo, privacy and blame. Long before the onset of HIV/AIDS, sexual practices had been colonised by concerns about immorality and fears about the consequences of moral decline in the political, public and private sphere.[14,15] The Victorian purity movement for example, with its well-rehearsed warnings against sex outside marriage, masturbation and homosexuality has been well documented.[15–18] Social action and sanctioning at the time served to perpetuate feelings of guilt and sin around any sexual expression outside the sanitised arena of marriage and procreation. As a result of this and many other examples, sexual health has regularly been subjected to degrees of silence over the years which have been difficult to overcome. This has contributed to the current situation where health researchers seeking to expand the pool of knowledge about the nature of human sexual experience and decision making have been hindered by the fact that the subject itself is still perceived as being 'not nice', too sensitive for objective research or unlikely to provide truthful responses.[19]

In the 1980s the emergence of AIDS and HIV as life-threatening conditions had a far-reaching impact on the need to discuss sexual activity and risk taking.[20] As a result of the devastating effects of HIV/AIDS experienced worldwide, sexual health issues were openly discussed beyond the parameters of epidemiology. Efforts were made to explore the causes, consequences and effects of sexual illness on an individual and at societal level.[21] Healthcare practice and research equally responded to the challenges arising from HIV/AIDS, recognising the consequences for patient care, infection control and professional health and safety amongst other issues.[8] However, while the emergence and worldwide recognition of the seriousness of HIV/AIDS was both effective and invaluable in bringing into the public arena the importance of research and discussion into sexual health, the success of the efforts made in HIV/AIDS reveal other silences.

The political climate in the face of the widespread hysteria around HIV in the early 1980s played a central role in the disease and to some extent sexual ill health, becoming established in the minds of the public as being far removed from the experiences of the white, male, heterosexual norm.[22] As a result gay men, black people, prostitutes and groups marginalised as 'other' were identified as the primary cause of HIV infection and harbourers of the disease.[13,23,24] Despite the progressive move towards wider consideration of sexual health called for by WHO in the 1970s, the effect of political attempts to manage the fear surrounding HIV/AIDS, by controlling sexual practices in the social and private spheres, resulted in a re-focussing on 'illness' as a consequence of poor sexual practices. The possibility of any other causative or influencing contextual factors on sexual health were lost in the impetus by politicians and media sources to create and recreate the divisions between 'us' and 'them' through the HIV tragedy, 'good' sex and health being again associated with morality and reunited with stoic versions of romantic love and duty.[25-27] Once historical parameters of good versus bad were erected around sexual behaviour and reinforced by the scientific 'proof' provided by HIV research, lifestyles which did not conform to the ideal were labelled 'unhealthy'. The practical effect of this labelling on individuals belonging to these marginalised groups is evidenced later in this book through chapters exploring the sexual health of black and minority ethnic men. This has also been highlighted in the literature in relation to the effects on other socially excluded or marginalised communities in the UK and worldwide.[22,28,29] However, with the emphasis of sexual-health work once again placed on prevention of the negative consequences of illness rather than promotion of health in any positive sense, what began as a public relations or harm-reduction exercise at parliamentary level also helped to confine the exploration of sexual health in its broadest sense.

The widespread and firm association of sexual health with HIV/AIDS has also to some extent developed into a belief that research into sexual health means HIV/AIDS research. Evidence of this was found in conducting the searches for literature review, during doctoral studies, by the plethora of research topics, funding and policies related specifically to HIV/AIDS research worldwide which were presented under the general title 'sexual health'. HIV/AIDS research is very well developed in both breadth and depth, receiving relatively large amounts of funding compared with other areas of sexual health from both private companies and public bodies.[6] The initial ring fencing of monies for research and development in this area and the efforts made by voluntary agencies in highlighting the effects of HIV-related illness means there exists a large number of both qualitative and quantitative studies relating specifically to HIV/AIDS.[29-32] While it can be argued that the HIV pandemic was, and still is, of major concern to all countries of the world, in Britain the concentration of sexual health research, funding and policies in this area has had negative consequences for sexual health research and policy development in general.

In Britain comparatively little funding or research attention in health has been paid to the sexual decision-making process and the preceding factors influencing patterns of sexual activity or sexual identity outside the parameters of HIV infection.[33] Research into sexual health in Britain in particular has furthermore focussed almost exclusively on minimising the effects of what are identified as poor sexual choices, with little consideration of how or why those choices take place. It could be argued that these things have been studied in relation to HIV and the results could be applied more generally to other sexual health situations.[1,34,35] However, it cannot be assumed that the same decision-making processes take place when the risks are not perceived to be life threatening.

Research evidence from more established areas, where the risk of death is well known as an outcome of particular health choices such as smoking, suggest that belief about actual risk of death acts as a modifying factor to behaviour.[36] This introduces the idea of perceived risk and impact on daily living as existing alongside real risk in health decisions. Issues relating to risk will be explored in different contexts throughout the other chapters.

Since the early 1990s attempts have been made by some sexual-health researchers and practitioners to provide a more holistic view of sexual health. There has been increasing recognition that simply recording infection rates and the numbers of unintended pregnancies was insufficient to bring about any change in the continued rise in sexually transmitted infections.[20,22,37,38] The issues raised by the WHO almost 20 years earlier had begun to be more widely and overtly promoted among sexual health specialists. To define sexual health solely in terms of a physical act or as a problematic activity is increasingly seen as denying the life-enhancing and positive aspects of sexual expression.[19,39] Attempts to define sexual health in care practice have therefore moved to incorporate a more holistic view of this concept rather than to try to confine it to a list of physical acts and their consequences. Such attempts do not remove, negate or minimise the importance of the physical aspects of sex, but seek to incorporate self-identity, emotional well-being and the ability to develop mutually satisfying relationships alongside physical expression as essential parts of any definition.[5,13,24]

Attempts to incorporate a multidimensional view of sexual health into healthcare policy and practice is problematic. Sexual health as a distinct area of care practice does not really exist. Sexual health is identified as incorporating a wide range of areas, including family planning, genito-urinary medicine (GUM) services and HIV/AIDS care. On closer inspection the scope of health policy and care service provision in these areas remain largely shackled to the physiological, stigmatised and fixed approaches to sexual health in the past. Sexual health education and training are not a compulsory part of healthcare professionals' basic training, and there are no standards relating to it on the core curriculum. The holistic approach to sexual health being encouraged through sexual health policy and research therefore effectively exists as a type of 'theoretical holism' which does not translate into practice. Sexual health continues to reflect a physiological focus with little or no general consideration given to the psychosexual aspects of care.[2] Research suggests that nurses, for example, find it hard to overcome their personal aversions to particular sexual practices or aspects of patient's sexuality and receive little or no training as to how to manage this, and this has a knock-on effect on the care they provide.[40]

Difficulties in delivering a holistic service are not confined to the individual healthcare practitioner. A healthcare professional's contribution to sexual healthcare occurs within a context where the sexual health services themselves are fragmented.[6] Sexual healthcare is thus delivered in a piecemeal fashion, with each service providing a portion of the care required without any real consideration of the whole. The provision of a fragmented healthcare service is not unique to sexual health; however, in sexual health the situation is compounded by the fact that many sexual health services and practitioners are unaware of whether or which other complimentary services are available.[41] As a result people are often left to search out and pursue additional services for themselves and so the quality of sexual healthcare varies immensely.

The tensions existing between the theories of sexual health, the realities of sexual health practice and the individual's experience make it difficult to select an effective definition of sexual health to use in this book. The WHO have acknowledged the difficulties in specifying the nature of sexual health and suggest that accepting the multifaceted nature of sexual health means that a single definition of a sexually healthy individual cannot exist.[42] As a result sexual health will not be defined absolutely in this book but will be seen as revolving around three broad concepts:

- The absence or avoidance of STIs and disorders affecting reproduction
- The control of fertility and avoidance of unwanted pregnancy
- Sexual expression and enjoyment without exploitation, oppression or abuse[11]

While Goldsmith's categorisation on sexual health is useful, it fails to adequately incorporate a number of key components which are important to later chapters that will explore the range of issues associated with the sexual health of men. The first issue is that of sexual identity. Sexual decisions incorporate recognition and acceptance of personal and group identities and the impact on the self and others in any sexual context. The third area of Goldsmith's categorisation indirectly refers to this when it talks of the need to avoid exploitation or oppression. However, this point needs to be incorporated much more explicitly to be of use to sexual policy makers, researchers or sexual health practice. Hendriks (1992), for example, includes in his definition of sexual health a view that it contributes to:

> The fulfilment of individual sexuality enabling a person to share this with consenting others without jeopardising the health and well-being of other persons.[43]

Hendriks suggests that this integrates a sense of responsibility in personal sexual identity and expression which ultimately translates into responsibility for the community as a whole, since the consequences impact at both an individual and societal level.[43] Practical examples of Hendriks' comments are reflected in the published epidemiological research indicating the social and individual health costs of high pregnancy rates and consequences of untreated STIs.[6,44] In these cases the impact of sexual decisions for the individual also has consequences for health and social care services due to the scale of the associated needs.

The linking of sexual health to the community highlights the importance of the social aspects of sexual health. Adopting the broad approach to sexual health outlined above in this study sees sexual health as involving much more than simply personal responsibility and includes the recognition that sexual health, particularly those aspects related to self-esteem and self-identity, not developed in isolation.[45] Helman[46] said that sexual health and the choices people make are influenced by their values, beliefs and concepts of self. As such, sexual health can be seen to reflect a person's experiences of socialisation and our environment.

This multidimensional view of sexual health allows research into the area to consider the possibility that individuals and groups may have different ideas about the nature of sexual health, as a result of their differing life experiences and viewpoints. Green and Tones[13] comment that sex and sexual activity have always been regulated by religion, state law or social pressure. As such it is difficult to discuss sexual health in isolation from individual life experiences. Like other aspects of life, once human experience and viewpoints are included, sexual health cannot be discussed, evaluated or provided for in a political and cultural vacuum.[13,43,46]

In this book the need to include a cultural and political understanding of the influences on the sexual health decisions of an individual or group is paramount. Without such an approach it will be impossible to provide any further insight, for example, as to why black Caribbean men consistently may appear at disproportionately higher risk of STIs,[20] or why erectile dysfunction may have consequences for families and communities as well as the individual men involved. Existing epidemiological data has been shown to be inadequate by itself to fully explain these issues. A contextual approach to the subject of men's sexual health is therefore necessary to promote understanding and for the development of strategies or services to optimise the health of men across all social groups.

In adopting a broader perspective on the issues concerning men and sexual health, the issues raised in this book will work towards fulfilling some of the requirements of the *National Strategy for Sexual Health and HIV* (NSSHH), published in 2001. This calls for researchers and others involved in sexual health to work to increase the British evidence base for provision of sexual health services and policy development.[6] The NSSHH identified research into sexual health as a basic requirement in initiating the strategies needed to assist sexual health services in bringing about changes in the sexual health profiles of all populations at risk of infection. Particular emphasis is placed in the NSSHH on research to facilitate understanding of:

- The sexual networks, health-seeking behaviour and risk behaviour of targeted groups
- The impact on ethnicity, deprivation and other socio-economic factors on sexual health (p. 45)

Many of the points raised in this book highlight the importance of understanding some of the wider social factors affecting behaviour and beliefs in relation to sex and sexual expression, and how they may impact on life choices and health. It is particularly important to identify the ways in which beliefs about sexual expression relate to both health decisions and individual perception of risk.

The importance of the broader context in which sexual decisions take place is influenced by the efforts taken in this book to include the practical and real-life situations in which men's sexual decisions occur. One of the issues pertaining to sexual health is the fact that individual knowledge and public belief systems often vary from what is scientifically proven or established through academic investigation. In all aspects of healthcare practice, both professional and lay definitions of health exist.[47,48] These are not necessarily distinct or wholly separate from each other, but may be confused, conflict or be a cause of misunderstanding. Sexual health, like other aspects of health, is open to interpretation and may be related to more general views about what it means to be healthy.[49] Therefore, despite the welcome changes made in academic and professional circles to see sexual health as a holistic and changeable concept, very little may have changed in the mind of the general public or sexual health professionals. Projects investigating sexual health issues among lay people and healthcare professionals, for example, have identified that individuals continue to associate sexual health solely with simply sexual intercourse and its consequences.[32,45,50]

In order to account for the range of issues described above, sexual health in this study is taken be a complex issue comprising the somatic, emotional, intellectual and social aspects of an individual.[51] Sexual health is accepted as being achieved when these characteristics positively interact.[42] As a concept there are many issues and experiences that are shared between human beings. However, the social influences on such things as sexual expression or acceptable sexual practices mean sexual health must also be recognised as a concept which changes over time both between groups and for individuals throughout the lifespan.[52]

In order to be able to research aspects of sexual health in detail using a contextual approach, it is important to narrow down the scope of the research to a specific group. The rest of this book will encourage the reader to debate and explore issues relating to the sexual health of men, the social group forming the main focus of this book.

The objective of Chapter 2 is to critically examine the impact of gender on the health of men. The authors are 'recasting masculinity' in an attempt to ensure that the reader is clear about the many perspectives influencing men, masculinity and health. In doing so they are able to suggest examples for developing public health approaches that will assist men in their future health decisions. It clearly sets the scene for the discussion to come in the remaining chapters and, in particular, Chapter 3. Chapter 3 explores the relationship between sexual health and the health of men. It incorporates a discussion of aspects of that relationship, including men's role in reproductive health and the effects of social, political and personal change on that role. This chapter will explore the challenges, constraints and opportunities for promoting positive sexual health in men.

Chapters 4 and 5 move from this wider view of the factors influencing men's health and their sexual health to begin to consider ill health. Physical ill health is examined in relation to STIs and the male-specific cancers of the prostate and testicles. Prostate cancer has been chosen as it is the most common cancer affecting men within the UK and one of the commonest worldwide. Testicular cancer has been chosen as it is the most common cancer affecting men in the 20- to 44-year-old age group, despite being a very uncommon cancer when compared with all cancers. This is followed by an examination of an often neglected area of sexual health: psychosexual care. Whilst exploring erectile dysfunction, it will also address links between psychological and physical sexual health and broader aspects of psychosexual care.

From ill-health issues, whether physical or psychosexual, the discussion moves on in Chapters 6 and 7 to explore the complexities of men's sexual behaviour. The discussion refers back to the definitions and perspectives examined in Chapter 2 in presenting a viewpoint from which to accept or challenge factors affecting sexual behaviours. It utilises condom use as an example to illustrate how some men make decisions about their own sexual activities and health-related risks, and highlights a need to understand the divisions that exist between male sexual identities in order to provide appropriate strategies for future sexual-health promotion. Chapter 8 demonstrates this clearly among a group of men who are frequently subjected to sexual and gender stereotyping. It reflects critically on the sexual health needs of men from black and minority ethnic groups, considering the reasons for the high levels of sexual ill health in this section of the population and suggesting ways forward in improving their health chances.

Finally, the content of this book will explore the important contributions made by statutory, voluntary and self-help organisations in providing effective sexual healthcare for men. It reviews the need for effective sexual healthcare in the light of current and contemporary health and social policy, and makes recommendations for developing sexual health services for men in a more gendered manner. It is important to remember that the book does not set out to provide the definitive argument for the sexual health and experiences of men, but hopes to encourage the reader to join with the contributors in raising questions and debating issues that will go some way to gaining a greater understanding of the sexual health of men.

REFERENCES

1 Crepaz N and Marks G. Towards an understanding of sexual risk behaviour in people living with HIV: a review of social, psychological and medical findings. *AIDS* 2002; **16**(2): 135–149.
2 Clifford D. Psychosexual awareness in everyday nursing. *Nurs Stand* 1998; **12**(39): 42–45.
3 Aggleton P and Tyrer P. Sexual Health. In: Whitly G, editor. *Learning about AIDS: scientific and social issues*. London: Churchill Livingstone; 1994.
4 Beacham S. Talking sex. *Nurs Stand* 1995; **10**(10): 56.
5 Royal College of Nursing. *Sexuality and sexual health in nursing practice*. London: Royal College of Nursing; 2000.
6 Department of Health. *The national strategy for sexual health and HIV*. London: Department of Health; 2001.
7 Fenton K and Wellings K. Sexual health and ethnicity. In: Shetty P, editor. *Heath and ethnicity*. London: Taylor and Francis; 2001. pp. 223–232.
8 Wilson H and McAndrews S, editors. *Sexual health – foundations for practice*. London: Baillière Tindall; 2000.
9 Stedman Y and Elsteen M. Rethinking sexual health clinics. *BMJ* 1995; **310**: 342–343.
10 Koshiti-Richmond A. The role of the nurse in promoting testicular self-examination. *Nurs Times* 1996; **92**(33): 40–41.
11 Goldsmith M. Family planning and reproductive health issues. In: Curtis H, editor. *Promoting sexual health*. London: BMA Foundation for AIDS; 1992. p. 121.
12 World Health Organization. *Education and treatment in sexuality: the training of health professionals*. Copenhagen: WHO; 1975.
13 Green J and Tones K. Sex and the world. In: McAndrews S, editor. *Sexual health: foundations for practice*. London: Baillière Tindall; 2000.
14 Beauviour S de. *The second sex*. Harmondsworth: Penguin; 1984.
15 Lancaster RN and Leonardo M di, editors. *The gender sexuality reader*. London: Routledge; 1997.
16 Masters WH, Johnson VE and Kolodny R. *Human sexuality*. New York: Harper Collins; 1995.
17 Bhabha HK. The other question: the stereotype and colonial discourse. In: Merck M, editor. *The sexual subject: a* Screen *reader in sexuality*. London: Routledge; 1992. Chapter 16.
18 Caplan P, editor. *The cultural construction of sexuality*. London: Tavistock Publications; 1987.
19 Pitts M. Sexual health. In: *The psychology of preventive health*. London: Routledge; 1996. pp. 67–81.
20 Adler MW. Sexual health – a health of the nation failure. *BMJ* 1997; **314**: 1743–1747.
21 Health Education Authority. *Health updated – sexual health*. London: HEA; 1994.
22 Hart G and Boulton M. Sexual behaviour in gay men: towards a sociology of risk. In: Hart G, editor. *AIDS risk: safety, sexuality and risk*. London: Taylor and Francis; 1995. pp. 55–67.
23 Department of Health. *HIV/AIDS and sexual health key area handbook*. London: Department of Health; 1993.

24 Harding J. *Sex acts*. London: Sage Publications; 1998.

25 Robinson N. The use of focus group methodology – with selected examples from sexual health research. *J Adv Nurs* 1999; **29**(4): 905–913.

26 Royal College of General Practitioners. *Health and prevention in primary care*. London: RCGP; 1981.

27 Sabo D and Gordon DF, editors. *Men's health and illness. Gender, power and the body*. London: Sage; 1995.

28 Valdiserri R. HIV/AIDS stigma, an impediment to public health. *Am J Public Health* 2002; **92**(3): 341–342.

29 Treicher P. AIDS, homophobia, and biomedical discourse: an epidemic of signification. In: Aggleton P, editor. *Culture, society and sexuality*. London: UCL Press; 1999. pp. 357–386.

30 Donenberg G, Emerson E, Bryant F, Wilson H and Weber-Shifrin E. Understanding AIDS risk behavior among adolescents in psychiatric care: links to psychopathology and peer relationships. *J Am Acad Child Adolesc Psychiatry* 2001; **40**(6): 642–653.

31 Holtzman D, Bland S, Lansky A and Mack K. HIV-related behaviours and perceptions among adults in 25 States: 1997 behavioral risk factor surveillance system. *Am J Public Health* 2001; **91**: 1882–1888.

32 Johnson A, Mercer C, Erens B, Copas A, McManus S, Wellings K, *et al*. Sexual behaviour in Britain: partnerships, practices and HIV risk behaviour. *Lancet* **358**(Dec): 1835–1842.

33 Adams J. Sex and politics. In: McAndrews S, editor. *Sexual health – foundations for practice*. London: Baillière Tindall/RCN; 2000. pp. 33–45.

34 Aggleton P, O'Reilly K, Slutkin G and Davies P. Risking everything? Risk behaviour, behaviour change and AIDS. *Science* 1994; **265**(5170): 341–345.

35 Cantana JA, Kegeles SM and Coates TJ. Towards an understanding of AIDS risk behaviour: An AIDS Risk Reduction Model (ARRM). *Health Educ Q* 1990; **17**(1): 53–72.

36 Woodland A and Hunt C. Healthy convictions. *Nurs Times* 1994; **90**(5): 32–33.

37 Bolton A. AIDS and promiscuity: muddles in the models of HIV prevention. *Med Anthropol* 1992; **14**: 145–223.

38 Taylor BM. Gender-power relations and safer sex negotiations. *J Adv Nurs* 1995; **22**(4): 687–693.

39 Williamson PR and Robinson S. Men's health: more than some of his parts. *Nurs Stand* 1999; **13**(18): 20.

40 Hayter M. Is non-judgmental care possible in the context of nurses' attitudes to patients' sexuality? *J Adv Nurs* 1996; **24**(4): 662–666.

41 Department of Health. *Effective commissioning of sexual health and HIV services*. London: DoH; 2003.

42 World Health Organization. *Concepts for sexual health*. Copenhagen: WHO; 1986.

43 Hendriks A. The political and legislative framework in which sexual health takes place. In: Curtis H, editor. *Promoting sexual health*. London: BMA Foundation for AIDS; 1992. pp. 155–166.

44 DiClemente R, Wingwood G, Crosby R, Sionean C, Cobb B, Harrington K, *et al*. Sexual risk behaviour associated with having older sex partners: a study of black adolescent females. *Sex Transm Dis* 2002; **29**(1): 20–24.

45 Merck M, editor. *The sexual subject: a* Screen *reader in sexuality.* London: Routledge; 1992.

46 Helman C. *Culture, health and illness.* London: Butterworth Heinemann; 1990.

47 McGee P. *Issues for transcultural nursing: a guide for teachers of nursing and health.* London: Chapman and Hall; 1992.

48 Valkimaki M, Suominen T and Peate I. Attitudes of professionals, students and the general public to people with HIV/AIDS: a review of the literature. *J Adv Nurs* 1998; **27**(4): 752–759.

49 Wilson T, Uuskula A, Feldman J, Holman S and Dehorvitz J. A case-control study of beliefs and behaviours associated with sexually transmitted disease occurrence in Estonia. *Sex Transm Dis* 2001; **28**(11): 624–629.

50 Rosenthal D and Moore SM. Stigma and ignorance: young people's beliefs about STDs. *Venereology* 1994; **7**(2): 62–66.

51 Lewis S and Bor R. Nurses knowledge of and attitudes towards sexuality and the relationship of these with nursing practice. *J Adv Nurs* 1994; **20**: 251–259.

52 Ewes S and Simnett I. *Promoting health – a practical guide to health promotion.* London: Scutari Press; 1993.

CHAPTER 2

Recasting masculinity: mapping out challenges and opportunities for public health

Graham Holroyd, Denise Richardson and James Webb

Key points

Defining masculinity.

Masculine identity and 'lifestyles'.

Masculine health inequalities.

Men's health-seeking behaviour.

Engendering and re-visioning social and health institutions and practice.

> From an early age we learn that the key to sexual difference lies in the make-up of men's and women's bodies. … A penis *means* masculinity or manhood, while breasts and vaginas denote femininity or womanhood. Common-sense ideas about sex differences also extend beyond the bounds of physical bodies to men's and women's psychological 'make-up' and patterns of behaviour. It is not unusual to hear people arguing that men are naturally the more aggressive sex, for example, or that women are much more emotional than men.[1] (p. 9)

But making a distinction between males and females implies that sexual or gender difference lies in the make-up of men's and women's bodies, and the development of conventional masculine and feminine behaviour. One of the most searching criticisms of gendered stereotyping comes in the form of Oakley's[2] claim that 'men are the real victims', alerting us to the fact that 'men [are] in crisis' (p. 76). This chapter focuses on 'Recasting Masculinity' and provides a critical review of a range of perspectives on the 'nature of masculinity'. Written in a clear and accessible style, it takes the reader on a journey illustrating the different ways in which these perspectives frame 'masculinity' and illuminates some of the problems for men's health and social well-being. The chapter will encourage the reader to consider the adequacy of various theoretical perspectives, including male liberationalists[3] as early as the 1970s arguing that men are victims of masculinity. The authors will argue that '*Gender* [Inequality] *on Planet Earth*'[4] is not a matter of individual wishes and choices, but is organised through social discourses, social institutions and social practices at all levels.

The authors also argue that in this century it is the men's movement that has the opportunity to negotiate a change in social thinking, politics and practice, because *Recasting Masculinity: Mapping Out Challenges and Opportunities for Public Health* questions our understanding of 'men' and 'masculinity', and the social structures which maintain gender inequalities and contribute to the crisis of masculinity that contributes to a form of 'manslaughter'. Indeed, all the perspectives and issues reviewed can be seen as developing a dialogue or debate in some way or another.

The UK government, through a plethora of policies, is committed to improving and positively promoting health. This it is undertaking, alongside tackling ill health and reducing health inequalities, by acknowledging the major socio-cultural and socio-economic causes of ill health. In doing so, the Government recognises that there is a direct link between poverty, social exclusion and ill health, all of which prevent individuals from accessing healthcare services and attaining optimum health. Improving health, narrowing the widening gap between rich and poor, and making health services more relevant to individual need is also a priority.[5] Of late, there have been a number of organisations and individuals advocating the fact that gender differences in healthcare and health status also need to be taken into account as another form of 'inequality', and that gender mainstreaming strategies, for policy and practice in healthcare delivery, should be adopted.[6] In the men's arena in particular, there have been noticeable and significant debates[7-10] regarding men's reluctance to access health services. It is therefore important to critically examine the impact of gender and masculinity on the health of men. In doing so, it is important to think laterally and develop a discussion about the way socially constructed barriers – the personal, social, economic and political factors, which are implicitly interwoven, on the one hand, and the ideas and practices relating to masculinity on the other, which is arguably important – underlie the central concern of recasting masculinity and preventing masculine health inequalities that may lead to mortality (slaughter of men) or 'manslaughter'.[4]

The interest in men's health has been steadily growing and initially came to the fore as relatively recently as 1992.[11] Other widely accepted health variables such as race and ethnicity, socio-economic status and geographical area had, by the 1970s, been joined by gender. The issue of gender then was seen to be increasingly important and had to be considered when explaining health: originating within the women's movement of the 1960s, differing from the earlier movement, with its emphasis on political representation,[12,13] and more concerned with 'sexual politics', critiques of domestic life,[14,15] personal relationships, psychological oppression,[16] women's responsibility for 'housework' and structure of femininity – some social forces which can make 'women sick'.[17] During this period, there was also an on-going growth in feminist research and the women's movement, contributing directly to the growth of knowledge and practice of the women's health movement.[18,19] In 1973, the first major text in this field, *Our Bodies Ourselves*, was published by the Boston Women's Health Collective. An edition was published in the UK in 1978, by Ackerman-Ross and Sochat.[20] Researchers and academics, however, still equated studies of gender and health almost exclusively with women. However, there were the minority of writers linking notions of masculinity and the male role with both physical and mental health issues. Doyal,[17] although considering only women's health initially, suggested that her findings might be used as a framework for change in health status and behaviour for men.

The growth of interest in men's studies in the 1980s brought into greater prominence questions about the relationship between concepts of health, masculinity, men's lives and their experiences of illness. The issue of masculinity, Watson[21] suggests, acknowledging the work of Sabo and Gordon,[19] is a complex interplay between the personal, social and political. However, as Oakley[4] suggests, men must 'take responsibility for what they are' (p. 220) if they are to seriously address the hazards of 'masculine lifestyles'.[22]

It could be argued that, to some men, 'ignorance is bliss' and they would rather not seek help.[23] This 'denial' or 'ignorance' which prevails among some men could prove to have further detrimental affects on their health, as this line of action generally increases the risk of the escalation of a health issue and could ultimately compromise its treatment or curability. This, it could be argued, is of particular significance in the arena of sexual health reflected in the Department of Health's (2001) *National Strategy for Sexual Health and HIV*.[24] Research has shown that male patients would generally be more willing to seek medical care – albeit curative – if such manifestations were enfeebling them, rather than to seek preventive care.[25] It needs to be made clear that there are many factors that prevent men from *actively* seeking regular health check-ups that can pose as barriers, and that other factors can act as barriers for men that prohibit their seeking treatment *after* diagnoses. For example, the *nature* of the disease that the male patient is diagnosed with could pose as a medical barrier post-diagnosis. Diseases such as male breast cancer and eating disorders may potentially have a 'social stigma'[26] attached to them. Although shared by men and women, these two illnesses have predominantly feminine relationships[27] and may lead to a very apathetic approach from men to seek treatment post-diagnosis. Men's 'failed health-seeking behaviour' is a by-product of damaging masculine dramaturgy[28] – a sociodrama:[2]

> ... games to which..., like [for] other men, are children's games – which are not seen for what they are because, precisely, the collective collusion [masculine domination] endows them with the necessity and reality of shared self-evidences.[29] (p. 75)

However, Bourdieu[29] also argues:

> ...that they have a double-edged privilege of indulging in the game of domination ... [but at the same time exposing] the desperate efforts of the 'child-man' to play the man and the childish despair into which his failures [here manifested as failed health or health-seeking behaviour] cast him. (p. 75)

Weltzin *et al.*[30] identified a belief held by some men that the treatment setting for such 'feminine diseases' is aimed at women,[31] such as the 'feminist treatment philosophy',[32-34] or that the treatment environment is feminised through discursive constructions of 'the eating disordered patient'[31] because of a significantly higher number of women forming the treatment group. However, research has suggested that 'all-male groups' may be worth considering so that men may also create a 'gendered space' wherein they can reflect on 'masculinity in crisis'[35] and take responsibility for what they are.[36] Then and only then can men as a group think about the way they behave; traditional and damaging notions of masculinity can be challenged and, to paraphrase Stoltenberg[35] in his *Refusing to be a Man*, men must live their lives in a way that will make a difference to themselves – transforming self[37] and developing health-protecting gendered behaviour.

Aspects of traditional notions of masculinity contribute to men's experience of their own health[10] and health issues. Meth and Pasick[38] suggest that masculinity is determined by physical, psychological and emotional development.[4,39] These, they argue, interact with societal and cultural expectations. Conversely, sex roles are biologically determined and understood in terms of anatomy, physiology and hormones; gender roles are constructed through psychological, cultural and social means.[40] A gender identity begins to take shape from birth, as soon as biological sex is determined and expectations designed to outline appropriate behaviour for each sex begin to be expressed. Stolenberg[35] agrees and argues that the notion of sexual identity is a fiction, a political and ethical construction with no basis in biology, which maintains destructive gender divisions and sexual injustice.

Gender identity includes psychosexual development, learning social roles and shaping sexual preferences. Social rearing, or socialisation, is a crucial element for gender identity. McCloskey[41] argues that:

> ... gender can be viewed as an accretion of learned habits, learned so well that they feel like external conditions, merely the way things are. It is a shell made by the snail and then confining it ... (p. xii)

Pressure to conform to prescribed roles comes from the family and is later re-enforced by peers, school, work and society as a whole. An important part of male gender identity is a fear of what is regarded as femininity, feminine values and feminine traits. It is said to be a common result of male socialisation and may lead to a 'loathing' of women and violence. Greer[42] warns that 'women don't know how much men hate them, when men hate them, or why'. (p. 280). Anthony Clare[36] agrees and admits that:

> ... all men, myself included, do not just love women ... We fear them, hate them, marginalize them, denigrate them and categorize them, and ... strive to control and dominate them. (p. 194)

As part of 'masculine identity' men 'talk about aggression' as a routine part of their life. The strange thing is that this 'masculine aggression' may be a much stronger predictor of self-destructive behaviour[4] and poor health for men.

From birth, boys generally are expected to be competitive, autonomous and independent and to suppress their emotions. Chodorow[43] suggests that social and economic status, race and ethnicity are all factors which affect the intensity of the messages from parents, and, for example, working-class fathers tend to be more insistent than middle-class fathers that their sons should adhere to sex-stereotyped roles. It is widely agreed that men in contemporary Western societies find it difficult to express their emotions adequately.[32] This emotional illiteracy, or failure to express emotions, in addition to the urge to be independent, could significantly influence men's health-related behaviour and ultimately their health status. Alongside other authors we would therefore suggest that men become good at 'non-speak' with regard to important emotional issues, and that it is regarded as a positive attribute to be emotionally invulnerable.[44] Men's resistance to acknowledging illness may be due, in part, to a fear of the dependence on women as carers. This contradicts the received wisdom that women are dependent on men. As Miller[3] has argued previously, it is women who are brought up to provide for the dependency needs of children, husbands and so on. Eichenbaum and Orbach[33] contrast the myth of men's independence with their actual reliance on women: boys can live with the expectation of continued maternal nurturance, first from their mother and later from their wife. At the same time as men acquire power in the outside world – by being born male in a patriarchal culture – they continue to be looked after (as children are) at home.

Marriage is good for men's health status; married males have lower death rates than those who have never married, and married men report better health than do single men. This suggests a possible 'health protecting' social support environment, provided by women. This may be due to the presence or absence of a significant female carer encouraging her male partner to seek help when needed and setting the tone for a 'healthy life'.[45] The idea that failing health signifies vulnerability may explain why some men will not admit to illness until it is too late. Men's denial of illness is so strong, argues Goldberg,[46] that it is one reason their average life span is considerably shorter than women's. Even pain as strong as a heart attack has been ignored, so that the victim would not be seen as weak or effeminate.

Employment will obviously affect health status. This being true for both women and men, though it may be that factors associated with paid employment and roles within the sphere of work, the public arena, are of special importance to men because of their socialisation to place a high value on success in work. Evans *et al.*[47] cite various authors who suggest numerous physical and emotional health problems, such as depression, irritability and insomnia, which can be attributed to loss of work. Over and above the direct effects of loss of income, unemployment in men can experience reduced self-esteem, autonomy and identity self-confidence that may contribute to the man's inability to cope with everyday problems. Generally, men in work enjoy better physical and mental health than those who are unemployed. Unemployment increases the risk of illness and premature death. A middle-aged man who loses his job is twice as likely to die in the following five years than a man who remains employed.[48]

Lorber and Farrell[40] suggest that men do not seek healthcare because of the socially gendered differences existing between men and women. To expand this point, there is strong evidence to suggest that there are profound differences between men's health and women's health,[17] the way in which they perceive health and health services and the different ways in which both sexes maintain their health. These differences suggest why the life expectancy for women in 2006 was approximately 81 years, whereas it was approximately 76 years for men. Life expectancy for both men and women is increasing; however, there is still a marked gender difference. This suggests that men do not enjoy as healthy a life as women, and that men would benefit greatly from regularly seeking healthcare and being actively involved in health education and health-promotion programmes throughout their lives. In the early 1900s, the gap between female and male life expectancy was 2–3 years in Western societies. By 2000, the gap had increased to 7–8 years in the same countries.[49]

Such hypotheses of men's shorter mortality rates relating to their lifestyles could instead be explained by physiological factors: women have a higher level of oestrogen in their bodies than men. This hormone is thought to act as an inhibitor against the onset of cardiovascular diseases.[50] Conversely, men boast a higher level of testosterone in their bodies. Although the testosterone hormone was essential in the prehistoric era for men to seek a mate and to aspire to be the 'alpha male', it is a male function that should possibly have been contributable only to the physicality of men's actions in the environment of evolutionary adaptation. However, testosterone still affects men's behaviour, and has been found to incite aggression and violence in men. This could explain the higher rate of premature deaths through 'risk-taking' and violent behaviours,[51] in comparison with women. This 'risk taking' behaviour may manifest itself, for example in 'risky' sexual behaviour, an assumption which correlates with Phillips'[50] findings. During adolescence, boys tend to put their health at risk by indulging in dangerous behaviour in keeping with their supposed machismo image. Boys have a higher rate of injury than girls from sports-related activities. Deaths from car accidents are proportionately higher amongst young adult males than in other groups of people,[52] and motor vehicle accidents are a leading cause of death for young males aged between 14 and 24 years. Over two-thirds of victims of violent crime are male, of whom 43% are assaulted on the street or in pubs.[11] It can be argued that men's life expectancy is shortened because of self-destructive tendencies developed at an early age. Men respond differently to stress and change than do women. As previously discussed, this is partly reflected in recent suicide trends. Suicide rates for males, during both adolescence and adulthood, are higher than those of females, which are steadily decreasing.[53] There is a worrying increase in suicide rates amongst young men.[11] This may be a reflection of men's unwillingness to solicit help when it is needed.[38] Through analysing epidemiological statistics of Canadian men's and women's mortality rates, Phillips found that male risk-taking behaviour seems to account for practically all excess mortality below 45 years of age. Phillips also found that men usually die from risk-taking behaviour before 60 years of age, and then tend to die from varying diseases after this age.

Sher[54] suggests that the different processes of socialisation and the different ways in which males and females are conditioned from birth could affect male and female occupational status and ultimately men's willingness to seek help. Through a longitudinal study of children, Sher found that the traditional male gender role was characterised by having aspirations for personal achievement, whereas girls' future objectives were to develop social and family relationships. It could be argued therefore that men would appear to be more sensitive to work stressors, achievements and failures, i.e. there is more pressure on them to perform in the public arena.[36,39,55] Furthermore, men's social status and identity are thought to be dependent on their working role and could therefore heighten pressure to maintain their occupation, and contribute, for example, to a more likely episode of a mental illness or mental ill-health.

White and Cash (2004), cited in Phillips,[50] suggest that male morbidity and mortality rates in Europe may be explained by the interplay of nature versus nurture, and this relationship may conspire to shorten the lifespan of men in contrast to women. Phillips'[50] findings are a discussion of Canadian mortality rates and may not be specific to Canadian socialisation issues and therefore not appropriate to men's behaviour and lifestyles in the UK. However, Renzetti and Curran[56] and Moon and Gillespie[57] suggest that the patterns in male behaviour, mortality and morbidity can be observed across *all* contemporary Western societies. It could be argued that the socialisation of men to pursue financial success does not create pressure, and instead it may be argued that a male's fixation on achievement may conjoin social gratification and appreciation with positive effects on identity and health.[58] Others will not necessarily face barriers that some men face.

Because men in the UK are representative of different classes and ethnicities, they can encounter a number of problems that can prevent them from actively seeking healthcare, be they sociological, financial, racially related or topical reasons. In essence, men are not a homogeneous group. Whitley[59] investigated the inequities that exist in Denver, USA, regarding black and Hispanic men's healthcare. Whitley found that men of these ethnic origins were not easily seeking healthcare because of a mixture of their own efforts and through factors not of their own doing. Of the men that Whitley interviewed, it was found that most of the men had a low socio-economic status, were in precarious employment, had a low educational attainment and displayed differing cultural norms and practices compared with the majority of Denver's male population. This illustrates how lack of money could pose as a barrier for some men actively seeking healthcare. Also, African-American men interviewed in Whitley's study told of political reasoning behind a poorer level of health among the male ethnic minorities of Denver, describing how some practices were not treating men of a low-income because it was not profitable to allocate resources for their needs. If there *was* such a lapse in governmental intervention, similarities could be made between Victorian England's 'laissez faire' approaches to healthcare,[60] although in this case race would be the issue rather than class. Because the UK does have a large number of ethnic minorities, it could be argued that Whitley's insights into how difficult men of an ethnic minority may find it 'hard to seek' healthcare could be useful in explaining racial and cultural barriers to men of ethnic minorities in the UK.

Some xenophobic men in the UK may not want to frequent their GP's surgery if they have 'racist' views and tendencies against the ethnicity of the GP, which may have been heightened in contemporary society. This could be the case as, out of the 34,000 GPs in Britain, approximately 5,000 that practice are from overseas. This form of racism – or racially related avoidance – should not just be expected to be one way, as a number of male patients from ethnic minorities may also not want to seek medical help from a Caucasian GP. They may prefer a GP of the same culture, possibly because of a belief that the terminology will be similar or easily recognisable. Language barriers may also be a reason for men of any ethnicity to seek medical help if the patient has difficulty in understanding the GP. Sexist or religious reasons could also pose as a problem for male patients. For example, if an Islamic male patient's GP is female, he may not be willing to be treated because of a number of prevailing religious beliefs regarding women. This is quite likely, as 38% of GPs in the UK are female.

The barriers that exist are not helped by an ignorance that appears to prevail throughout some institutions' and some medical professionals' views. A lack of knowledge, or 'gender-blindness' on a professional's or organisation's part, will affect the availability of resources to educate or to promote men's health. Cancer incidence and mortality are higher among men for almost all the cancers that affect both sexes.[47] This could be attributable to sex differences in modifiable risk factors such as alcoholism and smoking. Nevertheless, Evans *et al.*[47] found that 65% of women reported receiving instruction in breast self-examination, whereas only 10% of men revealed that they were taught testicular self-examination. A lower prevalence of self-examination in men could reveal gender biases in health practices. Interestingly, research has shown that small-scale efforts to educate men about testicular cancer have resulted in stronger intentions to self-examine, and an increased level of actual practice of self-examination. Striegel-Moore *et al.*'s research (2000), cited in Weltzin *et al.*,[30] found that men received less treatment than women (0.016%–0.140%) regarding intervention for eating disorders. This could be reflective of a political agenda – shaped by society's lack of knowledge that men can suffer from 'feminine' diseases such as eating disorders – that could favour the treatment of women over men in some or all diseases.

Evans *et al.*[47] have identified some reasons that might discourage health professionals from treating their male patients for testicular cancer:

- Concern about patient embarrassment
- Belief that testicular cancer is not a threat to adolescents
- Lack of time
- Unfamiliarity with technique
- The belief that testicular self-examination education is not part of a doctor's professional role

Evans *et al.*[47] also recognised a number of barriers that male patients can experience or can create themselves personally about testicular cancer:

- Not perceiving oneself to be at risk of cancer
- Practical and emotional barriers (for example, embarrassment or lack of time)
- Avoidant coping
- A failure to understand that the symptoms are potentially serious
- A fatalistic belief that nothing can be done in the event of a cancer diagnosis
- Perceptions that symptoms are transient
- Painful examination

Although these barriers are regarding testicular cancer, they could be applied to many other diseases that are pertinent to men. These apparent barriers are telling of institutional agendas that could be challenged.

Evans et al.[47] also postulate that lower levels of awareness of health concerns among men could correlate with a lack of media publicity. Katz et al. (2004), cited in Evans et al.,[47] found that media coverage of prostate and colorectal cancer (predominantly male cancers) is one-third of what is devoted to traditionally female cancers. This could mean that male health concerns have a relatively low profile. It is possible that the NHS does not support men's health initiatives as widely as it does those of women, as men seek relatively less medical help than women. Some feminists have the view that the NHS primarily serves the needs of men[6] and subordinates the needs of women as the wife and carer.[61] However, a lack of men's health may not correlate with the Department of Health's agendas and could be because of a number of other reasons, such as men's lifestyles.

Lifestyle is a nebulous concept. It may be described as a set of behaviours, undertaken by an individual or a group of people, which has an outcome.[62] Lifestyles can be defined as patterns of behavioural choices made from the alternatives that are available to people. They are therefore affected by their socio-economic status. Lifestyle for one individual is made up of the reactions and behaviour patterns that are learned through social interactions with parents, peers and siblings or through the influence of schools, the mass media, etc. Importantly, the term 'lifestyle' is often only used favourably, meaning *voluntary* choices people make. These may include alcohol consumption, dietary intake and how their leisure time is spent. However, there is overwhelming evidence of the need to acknowledge the importance of the economic and cultural dimensions that have a bearing on a person's lifestyle and over which the individual has little or no control.[56,62] However, Evans et al.'s[47] findings must not be considered representative of all health professionals' ways of working in the arena of men's health issues. It could be argued that the trend that Katz et al. (2004), cited in Evans et al.,[47] have identified is merely a vicious circle – requesting aid and seeking medical help conflicts with the stereotypical masculine gender role, characterised by strength and self-reliance, and so little intervention is made. Therefore, it is suggested that this seemingly impossible sequence of events compromises men's health.

The barriers that seem to threaten men's health status are, it is suggested, not solely men's responsibility. Other factors are thought to be at play. These might include institutional favouritism. It could be argued that the importance of men's health is subordinated by women's health and other varying factors that seem to conspire against the ease that some men *should* find in both seeking and experiencing good health and good healthcare. However, there do appear to be other reasons that men cannot or will not seek medical care. Some barriers have appeared to be more problematic for men than others. More research needs to be undertaken, in order to allow men's health to be more of a priority for men themselves and for both government-led and non-government-led initiatives to be developed. The actual causes of diseases and illnesses could be ascertained, articulated and addressed by men themselves, working collectively and in conjunction with healthcare providers, *before* men have to seek medical care. For example, the causes – and symptoms – of certain cancers could be made commonly understood in order to encourage men to attend for health screening. Health should no longer be assumed to be the responsibility of the health professional – all sectors of society could be involved in working together to educate men, promote men's health and ultimately to prevent disease. This could be undertaken throughout the lifespan of men, and through, for example, mass media campaigns, health education or consciousness-raising programmes, or through a sequence of more gender-sensitive, community-based initiatives. More effort could be made to increase attendance at health screening appointments, and raise awareness and understanding among all men in order that they may enjoy the benefits of early detection of symptoms of diseases, thus enabling healthcare professionals to treat these diseases and illnesses in the early stages. Although further research is needed in order to explain why women are more likely to visit the doctor than men, men must be encouraged to seek help (preventive as opposed to curative) as some men's knowledge of symptoms (for example, cancer warning signs) is poor, thus putting a number of men in greater danger through failing to understand the seriousness of these symptoms. Oakley[2] suggests a possible way for men by calling for a 'systems perspective' in addressing *Gender on Planet Earth*, arguing that:

> If on balance research shows, as it does, that women are more egalitarian than men, that they are less warlike and more interested in peace, and they are more aware of environmental issues, this is mostly because their experiences of life on earth remain qualitatively different from men's; they're still rooted in caring labour and personal relations. (p. 220)

The main problem is the personal, social, political, historical and environmental factors produced by a society predicated on an institutionalised system that creates gender inequality, which is making men sick. This chapter outlines a strategy of recasting masculinity and calls for men to take responsibility for what they are. The ambition has been to investigate the work of contributors in the men's arena, with and against the insights of feminists and contributors in the women's arena. What we see are theorists grappling with the contested nature of 'masculinity'. Together they comprise a re-visioning of the work from the men's arena, resulting in a shaking and loosening of the decisive logic of gender identities, thus providing an opening for interrogations of 'masculinity' and, implicitly, men's health. Helping men to gain control of their health ultimately involves their ability to develop 'their emotional literacy' and to carry out health-protecting behaviour through an awareness of healthier lifestyle choices. This chapter, hopefully, adds to the continuing debate regarding the ever-changing landscape of gender, masculinity and health, as Paglia[63] suggests:

> Maps for the future can be drawn only by those who have deeply studied the past. (p. 90)

REFERENCES

1 Edley N and Wetherall M. *Men in perspective: practice, power and identity*. Hemel Hempstead: Harvester Wheatsheaf; 1995.

2 Oakley A. The self and other dramas. In: Oakley A, editor. *Gender on Planet Earth*. Oxford: Blackwell; 2002a.

3 Miller SH. The making of a confused middle-aged husband. In: Pleck J and Sawyer J, editors. *Men and masculinity*. Englewood Cliffs, NJ: Prentice Hall; 1974.

4 Oakley A. Manslaughter. In: Oakley A, editor. *Gender on Planet Earth*. Oxford: Blackwell; 2002b.

5 Department of Health. *Choosing health: making healthy choices easier*. London: Department of Health; 2004.

6 Doyal L. *Integrating gender considerations into health policy development*. Brighton: WHO Regional Office Europe/European Men's Health Development Foundation; 2005.

7 Banks I. No man's land: men, illness and the NHS. *BMJ* 2001; **323**: 1058–1060.

8 Cameron E and Bernard J. Gender and disadvantage in health: 'men's health for a change'. In: Bartley M, Blane D and Davey Smith G, editor. *Sociology of health inequalities*. Oxford: Blackwell; 1998.

9 Holroyd G. Men's health in perspective. In: Jones LSM, editor. *The challenge of promoting health*. London: Macmillan/Open University Press; 1997.

10 Holroyd G. Silent cries – reflections on men's health promotion. In: Jones L, Sidell M and Douglas J, editors. *The challenge of promoting health – explorations and action*. Basingstoke: Macmillan/Open University Press; 2002.

11 Department of Health. *The state of the public health 1992*. London: Department of Health; 1993b.

12 Banks O. *Becoming a feminist: the origins of first wave feminism*. Sussex: Harvester Wheatsheaf; 1986.

13 Banks O. *Faces of feminism*. Oxford: Blackwell; 1993.

14 Rich A. *Of woman born: motherhood as experience and institution*. London: Virago; 1977.

15 Friedan B. *The feminine mystique*. Harmondsworth: Penguin; 1983.

16 Showalter E. *The female malady: women, madness and English culture 1830–1980*. London: Virago; 1987.

17 Doyal L. *What makes women sick?: Gender and the political*. London: Macmillan; 1995.

18 Doyal L. Health and the sexual division of labour: a case study of the women's health movement in Britain. *Crit Soc P* 1983; **3**(Summer): 21–33.

19 Sabo D and Gordon DF, editors. *Men's health and illness. Gender, power and the body*. London: Sage; 1995.

20 Ackerman-Ross FS and Sochat N. *Our bodies ourselves*. Boston: Boston Womens Health Collective; 1978.

21 Watson J. *Male bodies: health, culture and identity*. Buckingham: Open University Press; 2000.

22 Edwards T. *Cultures of masculinity*. London: Routledge; 2005.

23 Perelberg JR and Miller CA. *Gender and power in families*. London: Routledge; 1990.

24 Department of Health. *The national strategy for sexual health and HIV*. London: Department of Health; 2001.

25 Oliffe J and Mróz L. *Men interviewing men about health and illness: ten lessons learned*. British Columbia: University of British Columbia, Canada; 2005.

26 Goffman E. *Stigma: notes on the management of spoilt identity*. Englewood Cliffs, NJ: Prentice Hall; 1964.

27 Malson H. Anorexic bodies and the discursive production of feminine excess. In: Ussher JM, editor. *Body talk: the material and discursive regulation of sexuality, madness and reproduction*. London: Routledge; 1997.

28 Goffman E. *The presentation of self in everyday life*. New York: Doubleday Anchor; 1959.

29 Bourdieu P. *Masculine domination*. Oxford: Polity Press/Blackwell; 2001.

30 Weltzin TE, Weisensel N, Franczyk D, Burnett K, Klitz C and Bean P. *Eating disorders in men: update*. Wisconsin: Medical College of Wisconsin; 1998.

31 Malson H, Finn DM, Clarke S and Anderson G. The eating disordered patient: a discourse analysis of accounts of treatment experiences. *J Community Appl Soc Pyschol* 2004; **14**(6): 473–489.

32 Eichenbaum L and Orbach S. *Understanding women: a feminist psychoanalytic account*. Harmondsworth: Penguin; 1982.

33 Eichenbaum L and Orbach S. *Understanding women*. Harmondsworth: Penguin; 1985.

34 Stein J. *Empowerment and women's health: theory, methods and practice*. London: Zed Books; 1997.

35 Stoltenberg J. *Refusing to be a man: essays on sex and justice*. London: UCL Press; 2000.

36 Clare A. *On men: masculinity in crisis*. London: Chatto and Windus; 2000.

37 Giddens A. *Modernity and self-identity: self and society in the late modern age*. Cambridge: Polity; 1991.

38 Meth RL and Pasick RS. *Men in therapy, the challenge to change*. New York: The Guildford Press; 1990.

39 Greer G. Masculinity. In: Greer G, editor. *The whole woman*. London: Doubleday; 1999a.

40 Lorber J and Farrell SA. *The social construction of gender*. London: Sage; 1991.

41 McCloskey DN. *Crossing*. Chicago: University of Chicago Press; 1999.

42 Greer G. Loathing. In: Greer G, editor. *The whole woman*. London: Doubleday; 1999b.

43 Chodorow N. *The reproduction of mothering psychoanalysis and the sociology of gender*. Berkeley: University of California Press; 1978.

44 Holroyd G. A tentative look at men's health. *Men Too* 1990(Autumn): 5–7.

45 Miles A. *Women, health and medicine*. Milton Keynes: Open University Press; 1991.

46 Goldberg H. *The hazard of being male*. New York: New American Library; 1976.

47 Evans R, Brotherstone H, Miles A and Wardle J. *Gender differences in early detection of cancer*. London: University College London; 2004.

48 Department of Health. *Saving lives: our healthier nation.* London: Department of Health; 1999.

49 Sadler C. DIY male maintenance. *Nurs Mirror* 1985; **160**(12): 16–19.

50 Phillips SP. *Risky business: explaining the gender gap in longevity.* Kingston, Ont: Queen's University; 2004.

51 Vaarenen H. Speeding boys and the romance of destruction. Nordic Institute for Women's Studies and Gender Research. *NIKK Magasin* 2005; **3**(2005): 42–45.

52 Sarafino EP. *Health psychology.* London: Wiley; 1990.

53 Charlton J. Suicide trends in England and Wales: trends in factors associated with suicide deaths. *Population Trends* 1993. Report No. 71.

54 Sher L. *Per capita income is related to suicide rates in men but not in women.* New York: Columbia University; 2005.

55 Oakley A. *Sex, gender & society.* Melbourne: Temple Smith; 1972.

56 Renzetti CM and Curran DJ. *Women, men and society.* Boston: Allyn and Bacon; 1995.

57 Moon G and Gillespie R. *Society and health: an introduction to social science for health care professionals.* London: Routledge; 1995.

58 Winkler D, Pjrek E and Kasper S. *Gender-specific symptoms of depression and anger attacks.* Vienna, Austria: Medical University of Vienna; 2005.

59 Whitley EM, Samuels BA, Wright RA and Everhart RM. *Identification of barriers to healthcare access for underserved men in Denver.* Denver, CO: Denver Health, Community Voices; 2002.

60 Baggott R. *Public health: policy and politics.* New York: Palgrave; 2000.

61 Naidoo J and Wills J. *Health promotion: foundations for practice.* Oxford: Harcourt; 2002.

62 Blaxter M. *Health and lifestyles.* London: Routledge; 1990.

63 Paglia C. *Sex, art and American culture.* London: Penguin; 1992.

CHAPTER 3

Men and sexual health

Laura Serrant-Green

Key points

Men's sexual health remains marginalised within research, policy development and service provision around sexual health.

Men's health is predominantly associated with physical functioning and reproductive ability.

A more holistic approach to research, policy and service delivery is needed in order to advance the sexual health of men.

This chapter will explore the relationship between sexual health and the health of men. It incorporates a discussion of different aspects of that relationship including gender inequality in sexual health work, men's role in reproductive health and the effects of social, political and personal change on that role. This chapter will explore the challenges, constraints and opportunities for promoting positive sexual health in men and provides a broad context for some of the discussions to follow in later chapters.

The introduction to this book highlighted some of the ways in which much of the research evidence on sexual health, particularly in the UK, is unequally distributed in favour of studies into HIV/AIDS. However, when we consider the range of information published relating to sexual health subjects in general, another area of concern is revealed – that of gender inequality. Unlike many other areas of society, focussing on the issue of gender bias in sexual health research and information production reveals that the male as the subject of the information available is relatively absent. Until the early 1990s comparatively little had been published in relation to men's sexual health and the need to provide appropriate male-centred services.[1,2] Until that time, particularly in the UK, the views, needs and voices of men as gendered subjects in sexual health were conspicuous by their absence. In general, research and other studies into sexual health and gender meant researching women's health.[3]

The roots of the disparity between the association of men and women with sexual health are longstanding. To some extent they may be explained by considering the historical and political contexts in which sexual health policy, service planning and provision takes place. Historically the sanctioning of sexual practices, behaviour and sexuality in Britain has traditionally been closely associated with control of the sexual expression of women.[4] Attempts to control the sexual activities of the public were, to a great extent, centred on the sanctioning of female sexual behaviour through public pressure, policy and criminal law. Much has been written illustrating the ways in which British society worked to criminalise and pathologise female sexual expression to a greater extent than male sexual practices.[5–8]

At a time when medicine was perhaps one of the great controlling factors in British society, the pathologising of female sexual practice meant it could be opened up to scrutiny by the medical profession and society as a whole in an attempt to control it.[4] While the methods used to control sexual expression in women were at times abhorrent and damaging, the push to control women's sexual practices worked to cement the belief that any association between gender and sexual health concerned women's health.[9,10] The continuation of sexual health promotion approaches based on these beliefs, even into the twenty-first century, is partly responsible for the situation today where for the vast majority of the public seeking to understand 'gender and sexual health' means focussing on 'women and sexual health'. To some extent therefore it could be argued that men are not readily identified as subjects of research, policy and service development in sexual health because historically and politically their behaviour has not been pathologised.

The issue of inequality relating to the relationships between men, women and sexual health go beyond simply the frequency of the associations. In criticising the poor levels of provision of information and lack of support for men's sexual health issues, men's health organisations have also commented on the restrictive approach taken by researchers and service providers to the sexual health needs of men.[11,12] In conjunction with the lack of research studies into men's sexual health, it is evident that a wider variety of approaches is taken in relation to the sexual health of women.[2] The range of subjects covered in female-centred studies and policies in sexual health vary from pure information-giving to a wider exploration of the psychosocial issues related to the sexual health needs of women, service development and how to seek further help or support. In contrast, the resources and services specifically produced for men are predominantly identified as focussing on the physiological aspects of men's sexual identity and, unlike those for women, less likely to incorporate a multidimensional approach.[13] In relation to sexual health practice, policy and service development therefore, even when men's issues are considered, this is frequently constrained to incorporating the physical aspects of sexual expression and the illnesses and diseases associated with poor sexual choices. In the main, little or no consideration is given to the psychological and social impact of these conditions on men's lives.[9]

It is important to note that the recent notable exception to this is the attention given to male erectile dysfunction following the launch of sildenafil citrate (Viagra) onto the UK market in September 1998. In one sense the publicity given to erectile dysfunction did, as usual, focus on the physical aspects of male sexual functioning. However, the launch of Viagra was significant, because it not only signalled a change by primarily highlighting men's sexual health but appeared to initiate open discussion of the psychosocial impact of the consequences of poor sexual health on men. However, like the earlier attention given to HIV, the contexts in which the benefits of Viagra emerged to be incorporated into discussions of men's sexual health contain cautionary notes. Viagra, its efficiency in treating erectile dysfunction and the possible benefits for men's sexual health emerged as a bi-product of using the drug as a treatment for hypertension, for which it was originally designed.[14] While the discovery of additional benefits of a drug for other conditions is not unique, the mass publicity given to Viagra led to increased demands for the product.[15]

The emergence of this drug occurred against a historical backdrop of a lack of information about men's health. This makes it difficult to surmise whether the increased demand for Viagra and the associated rise in public awareness of the psychosocial problems of erectile dysfunction in men were the result of a hidden problem or the publicity surrounding the 'miracle' effects of the drug. In either case the links between a notable increase in the diagnosis of erectile dysfunction, the restrictions placed on its distribution by the UK government and the large revenues generated for the drug company producing it have since been subjects of continuing debate in political, medical and media circles.[16] The silences encased within the debates around Viagra include the way in which political and social reactions to this drug have progressively equated it with epitomising the notion of men's sexual health. In doing so the exposure and open discussion of the personal and emotional costs of sexual ill health in men which were enabled through the launch of Viagra were juxtaposed by a refocussing of the male sexual health agenda around physical prowess.

The disparity in the availability of information and research between men and women within a wider health context is not exclusive to issues of sexual health but is part of a general trend. Researchers into men's health and support groups argue that men's health in general is an area of unmet need that has dire consequences on the quality and quantity of life of the modern man.[17,18] Medical sociologists and health professionals have begun to highlight the discrepancy between the health education and information produced for men compared with women. They comment for example that, despite an increase in the application of initiatives to improve health across the population in Britain, middle-aged men are rarely receiving any preventative healthcare.[19] This is reinforced by other researchers who point out that, unlike women's health and strategies aimed at the public in general, provision for men's health has not progressed sufficiently from the treatment of ill-health models of the past.[1,9,18]

The implications of the hidden aspects of male sexual health and the lack of reaction to it as an area of health need must be appraised in the light of the gender bias in society. The marginalised positioning of men as subjects of sexual health research is strange, because historically and politically in many societies men, and white, middle-class heterosexual men in particular, have been centralised as the norm. However, as discussed earlier, in sexual health the positions in relation to gender are reversed, with women's sexual health occupying the 'dominant' position. While on the one hand the silence denoted by men and sexual health as a subject may be a reflection of inequality in a society that overtly and covertly identifies male sexual expression as unproblematic, the outcomes are not necessarily beneficial to the sexual health of men.[17]

In identifying male heterosexual activity as normal, society and history has worked to silence the broader range of needs associated with it. The consequences for heterosexual men are reflected in their relative absence from research, policy and service development in sexual health, particularly that concerning preventative health and community-based support.[13] The magnitude of the silences brought about by this situation increase when consideration is given to the types of sexual health information produced on HIV prevention since the advent of AIDS. The sexual health information provided exclusively for males in relation to HIV prevention and promotion of safer sex practices is predominantly geared to the needs of gay and bisexual men.[20] Here too the label of normality impressed upon heterosexual male sexuality works to simultaneously render it absent from the main focus of research, policy and service development in sexual health, while further marginalising the sexual behaviour of gay and bisexual men. The lack of publicity given to heterosexual male sexual behaviour is a matter of grave concern, since reports indicate that heterosexual transmission rates for HIV in the new millennium are now rising at a faster rate than that of homosexual transmission.[21] Despite this, it seems that sexual health and its consequences are still being identified by politicians, health information and service providers as predominantly an issue for men who have sex with men, rather than the exclusively heterosexual male.

The above discussion illustrates how the historical and political contexts in which the emerging sexual health issues are determined is less likely to identify men, and heterosexual men in particular, as the target group. In the light of this it is pertinent to consider whether women have a greater need for preventative sexual health information and services than their male counterparts. This was investigated in one of my previous studies,[22] which considered whether women were at greater risk of sexually related illness as indicated by a number of health-related factors, including incidence rates for sexually transmitted infections (STIs) and male participation in potentially risky activity.

The consequences of unprotected sex are well documented. These include the increased HIV transmission risk and the associated reduction in the life expectancy of both partners, as well as the possibility of STI transmission affecting quality of life and fertility.[23-25] In research conducted at various genito-urinary medicine (GUM) clinics across Britain, men in all ethnic groups are consistently reported to have a higher incidence of diagnosed STI than women from the same groups.[26,27] Studies from outside Britain also show a similar pattern of infection along gender lines and support the suggestion that greater sexual risk among men may be a worldwide issue rather than simply an isolated issue.[28,29] The consistency of the disparity in infection rates across socio-economic groupings, ethnicities and even geographical boundaries raises the question 'Why?'.

Health and life chances are affected by a whole host of issues spanning the socio-economic, genetic and contextual situation of the individual as well as their perception of the risks associated with a particular activity.[30,31] However, although there are varying views as to its effectiveness, it is also accepted that the level of knowledge an individual has concerning the risks involved in a particular activity plays some part in their decision to continue or change potentially risky behaviours.[32] Despite the high rates in STI in men and the growing recognition of their psychosocial needs in relation to sexual health, there are relatively few men-only or male-focussed sexual health centres[11]. With the exception of GUM clinics, sexual health services in many countries are identified as encompassing family planning clinics, local health centres and maternity services, developing which predominantly sustains a continuous link with women throughout their reproductive life.[33] In contrast, men's sexual health provision by statutory health services, where it exists, takes place 'after the fact' in treating sexual infection or urological disorders. Prevention or proactive promotion of men's sexual health in general occurs as an additional or compounding concern to women's health, particularly in relation to fertility and family planning.

Reviews of past approaches to family planning and fertility services reveal a lack of focus on the male perspective beyond the need to use condoms or provide the quality and quantity of sperm required for successful conception. The role of the male appeared to be constrained and confined once again to the ability to contribute to procreation or the lack of it. Men's health groups and political lobbies have evolved greatly since the mid-1990s to advance the broader needs of men across the spectrum of the reproductive cycle including the arenas of child care, family services and involvement in caring sexual relationships throughout their lifespan. Many of these organisations came together in 2002 to launch the International Men's Health Week and the associated International Men's Health Database on the Internet. These are important developments as they have begun to reset the landscape of men's sexual health within a broader context of men's general health needs, which includes the social, psychological and physical aspects of men's lives.

Health education approaches to sexual health are based on a view that a lack of accurate and appropriate information reduces the individual's ability to exercise free will in making informed choices within the contexts of their individual situation.[34] In relation to sexual health, this view is challenged by research which demonstrates that, despite information about sexual risk reduction being widely available since the 1980s, infection rates for sexually transmitted infections continue to rise.[24] The ineffectiveness of relying on information alone to bring about improvements in health is highlighted by a range of researchers, who point to the need to consider the wider contexts in which health is maintained and any information provided is interpreted.[35,36] When this information is coupled with the lack of a broad sexual health focus on men in the practice arena, the higher rates of sexual ill health in males is not surprising.

In some cases the high incidence rates of sexually related disorders amongst men could be considered to be associated with the social aspects of the male experience in society. Sabo and Gordon[1] reported that the leading causes of death in males were as a result of their behaviours. They identified that masculinity was a defining factor in considering risk and men's health, and also acted as a barrier to men developing a consciousness or seeking help in relation to their health. The socialising of many men into societies which prescribes that men are strong, unemotional and unconcerned with family life may therefore encourage individual behaviours which compromise men's sexual health.

In general health data, men have been reported as being more likely to delay in seeking medical advice when they are ill[37,38] and often denying their symptoms.[2] It has also been shown that men have a greater tendency to participate in activities which present risks to their health, such as excessive alcohol and tobacco consumption,[13,38,39] have an unhealthy diet[3] and follow a sedentary lifestyle.[2] The higher incidence of alcohol and drug use in men[19] may be considered as adding to the potential sexual health risks when viewed alongside reports which indicate that use of alcohol has an uninhibiting effect on sexual behaviour.[40–42] This is reflected in the higher incidence of reported unsafe sexual practices under the influence of alcohol and other drugs.[23]

The majority of sex-related health issues are preventable and easily managed or treated if detected early.[8] Historically based, stereotypical views of masculinity and sexual health in Britain, however, which reinforce an engendered belief that sexual illness is associated with 'women's problems', are unlikely to encourage men to adopt a proactive approach to their sexual health. This may go some way to explaining the low use of prevention advice services by men and their higher risk of many preventable diseases.[13,43] In order to begin to bring about a behavioural or attitudinal change in relation to sexual health, what must be determined are the factors which impact on or influence the sexual-health decisions of men in particular situations.

Many of the studies highlighted above provide important quantitative data to illustrate the need to include men as well as women in strategies to improve the sexual health of the public. However, without greater insight into how and why men are at risk with regard to their sexual health, it is impossible to determine what form any action should take and whether it is achievable. What is required is a gendered approach to research, policy and service development in men's sexual health. This means attempting to identify and understand the factors influencing the sexual health-seeking and risk-taking activities of men in the context of their life experiences and socio-cultural positioning. This will enable researchers, policy makers and sexual health service providers to appraise men's sexual health and decisions about their health-related activities in light of their particular social, cultural and individual experiences rather than despite them.

The relative lack of knowledge about the multidimensional nature of male sexual health and sexual expression hampers the development of any services or initiatives to address the challenges posed by men's sexual health.[44] In order to progress the work into men's sexual health, it is desirable to produce research, policies and sexual health services aimed at more than monitoring the physical consequences of male sexual practices.[12,17,45] The magnitude of the silences around men's sexual health is produced as a result of the lack of insight into the broader contexts of men's sexual lives for research studies, policy and service developments that acknowledge the physical basis of male sexual expression but are not constrained or defined by it. Research, policy and sexual health services must therefore incorporate the psychological, social and cultural aspects of men's sexual health in order to produce the information sources for the development of further research and health-promotion strategies.[18]

This wider approach to the sexual health of men is reinforced by the strategic direction of the World Health Organization (WHO) in its sexual health agenda. The WHO acknowledges that addressing sexual health requires understanding and appreciation of sexuality, gender roles and power in designing and providing services.[46] Their agenda for sexual health recognises that achieving positive sexual health for men and women includes pleasure and responsibility as well as physical functioning, in order to promote understanding of sexuality and its impact on practices, partners and reproduction.

CONCLUSION

This chapter has introduced many areas for discussion relating to the marginalisation of men as the subject of sexual health research, policy and service provision. It has also highlighted a need to broaden the view of men's sexual health beyond the purely physical to encompass a more holistic perspective. Incorporating this holistic perspective on men's sexual health brings with it challenges as well as opportunities to researchers, policy makers and service providers. Success is dependent on a number of competing issues such as ensuring the validity of data collection, given researcher bias, political pressures and difficulties in discussing such a private and sensitive issue. Research, policy development and service provision in men's sexual health cannot achieve any real progress towards a holistic approach unless it goes beyond concerns related to behaviour, numbers of partners and practices, to the underlying social, cultural and economic factors that underpin an individual's sexual health behaviour, makes them vulnerable to risks, and affects the ways in which sexual relationships are sought, desired and experienced by men. To do this does not mean rejecting past information or negation of the physical aspects of men's sexual health. Instead it encourages researchers, policy makers and service providers to introduce alternative, evidence-based holistic viewpoints to the knowledge gained from the field of STI/HIV prevention and care, gender studies and family planning, among others.[46] Failure to engage with this holistic perspective on men's sexual health will continue to hamper efforts to effectively understand and provide for the complex sexual health needs of a significant proportion of society.

REFERENCES

1 Sabo D and Gordon DF, editors. *Men's health and illness. Gender, power and the body.* London: Sage; 1995.
2 Watson J. *Male bodies. Health, culture and difference.* Buckingham: Open University Press; 2000.
3 Fareed A. Equal rights for men. *Nurs Times* 1994; **90**(5): 26–29.
4 Lancaster RN and Leonardo M di, editors. *The gender sexuality reader.* London: Routledge; 1997.
5 Master WH, Johnson VE and Kolodny R. *Human sexuality.* New York: Harper Collins; 1995.
6 Parker R and Aggleton P, editors. *Culture, society and sexuality. A reader.* London: UCL Press; 1999.
7 Merck M, editor. *The sexual subject: a screen reader in sexuality.* London: Routledge; 1992.
8 Wilson H and McAndrews S, editors. *Sexual health – foundations for practice.* London: Baillière Tindall; 2000.
9 Williamson PR and Robinson S. Men's health: More than some of his parts. *Nurs Stand* 1999; **13**(18): 20.
10 Verbrugge LM. Gender and health: an update on hypothesis and evidence. *J Health Soc Behav* 1985; **26**: 156–182.
11 Brown I and Lunt F. Evaluating a 'well man' clinic. *Health Visitor* 1992; **65**(1): 12–14.
12 Ions V. The trouble with men. *Nurs Stand* 2000; **14**(34): 61.
13 Luck M, Bamford M and Williamson P. *Men's health: perspectives, diversity and paradox.* Oxford: Blackwell Science; 2000.

14 Shakir SAW, Wilton LV, Boshier A, Layton D and Heeley E. Cardiovascular events in users of sildenafil: Results from first phase of prescription event monitoring in England. *BMJ* 2001; **322**: 651–652.

15 Kaye JA and Jick H. Incidence of erectile dysfunction and characteristics of patients before and after the introduction of sildenafil in the United Kingdom: cross sectional study with comparison patients. *BMJ* 2003; **326**: 424–425.

16 Ralph D and McNicholas T. UK management guidelines for erectile dysfunction. *BMJ* 2000; **321**: 499–503.

17 Lee C and Owens G. *The psychology of men's health*. Buckingham: Open University Press; 2002.

18 O'Dowd T and Jewell D, editors. *Men's health*. Oxford: Oxford University Press; 1998.

19 Robertson S. Men's health promotion in the UK: a hidden problem. *Br J Nurs* 1995; **4**(7): 399–401.

20 Treicher P. AIDS, homophobia, and biomedical discourse: an epidemic of signification. In: Aggleton P, editor. *Culture, society and sexuality*. London: UCL Press; 1999. pp. 357–386.

21 Department of Health. *The national strategy for sexual health and HIV*. London: Department of Health; 2001.

22 Serrant-Green L. *Black Caribbean men, sexual health decisions and silences*. PhD Thesis. Nottingham: University of Nottingham; 2004.

23 Health Education Authority. *Health updated – sexual health*. London: HEA; 1994.

24 Adler MW. Sexual health – a health of the nation failure. *BMJ* 1997; **314**: 1743–1747.

25 Buve A, Laga M and Piot P. Where are we now? Sexually transmitted diseases. *Health Policy Plan* 1993; **8**(3): 277–281.

26 Fenton K, Korovessis C, Johnson A, McCadden A, McManus S, Wellings K, *et al.* Sexual behaviour in Britain: reported sexually transmitted infections and prevalent genital *Chlamydia trachomatis* infection. *Lancet* 2001; **358**(Dec): 1851–1854.

27 Hughes G, Brady A, Catchpole M, Fenton K, Rogers P, Kinghorn G, *et al.* Characteristics of those who repeatedly acquire sexually transmitted infections: A retrospective cohort study of attendees at three urban sexually transmitted disease clinics in England. *Sex Transm Dis* 2001; **28**(7): 379–386.

28 Donenberg G, Emerson E, Bryant F, Wilson H and Weber-Shifrin E. Understanding AIDS risk behaviour among adolescents in psychiatric care: links to psychopathology and peer relationships. *J Am Acad Child Adolesc Psychiatry* 2001; **40**(6): 642–653.

29 Ford K and Norris AE. Sexually transmitted diseases: experience and risk factors among urban, low income, African American and hispanic youth. *Ethn Health* 1996; **1**(2): 175–184.

30 Fonck K, Mwai C, Ndinya-Achola J, Bwayo J and Temmerman M. Health-seeking and sexual behaviours among primary healthcare patients in Nairobi, Kenya. *Sex Transm Dis* 2002; **29**(2): 106–111.

31 Conner M and Norman P, editors. *Predicting health behaviour*. Buckingham: Open University Press; 1998.

32 Lupton D. *Risk*. London: Routledge; 1999.

33 Davidson N and Lloyd T, editors. *Promoting men's health: a guide for practitioners*. London: Baillière Tindall; 2001.

34 Woodland A and Hunt C. Healthy convictions. *Nurs Times* 1994; **90**(5): 32–33.

35 Lomas J. Social capital and health: Implications for public health and epidemiology. *Soc Sci Med* 1998; **47**(9): 1181–1188.

36 Gillies P. The effectiveness of alliances and partnerships for health promotion. *Health Promotion International* 1998; **13**: 1–21.

37 Royal College of Nursing. *Survey of district directors of public health*. London: RCN; 1995.

38 Platzer H. Ageing in men and the crisis of middle age. *Nursing* 1988; **26**: 963–965.

39 Williamson P. Their own worst enemy. *Nurs Times* 1995; **48**(4): 24–27.

40 Aggleton P, O'Reilly K, Slutkin G and Davies P. Risking everything? Risk behaviour, behaviour change and AIDS. *Science* 1994; **265**(5170): 341–345.

41 Ford K, Sohn W and Lepkowski J. American adolescents: sexual mixing patterns, bridge partners and concurrency. *Sex Transm Infect* 2002; **29**(1): 13–19.

42 Geringer WM, Marks S, Allen WJ and Armstrong KA. Knowledge, attitudes and behaviour related to condom use and STDs in a high risk population. *J Sex Res* 1993; **30**(1): 75–83.

43 Mac an Ghaill M. *The making of men. Masculinities, sexualities and schooling*. Buckingham: Open University Press; 1994.

44 Petersen A. *Unmasking the masculine. Men and 'identity' in a sceptical age*. London: Sage; 1998.

45 Harrison T and Dignan K, editors. *Men's health: an introduction for nurses and health professionals*. London: Churchill Livingstone; 1999.

46 World Health Organization 2003. Gender and reproductive rights. Retrieved 04/12/03 from http://www.who.int/reproductive-health/gender/sexualhealth.html

CHAPTER 4

Physical sexual ill health

John McLuskey and Laura Serrant-Green

Key points

Sexual ill health is not equally distributed across the male population.

Sexually transmitted infections have continued to increase since 2000, but they are easily treatable in most men.

Incidence of prostate cancer has been increasing across all male groups, but this may not be a true increase. However, the disease has always been more common in black African-Caribbean men.

Whilst it is specifically a male-only cancer, it is important to remember that testicular cancer is rare.

INTRODUCTION

This chapter provides an overview of some of the major challenges to men's physical sexual health in the twenty-first century. This is an important aspect of understanding the sexual health of men, as the physical aspects of men's sexuality and sexual behaviour are often placed at the centre of their sexual identity. There are many ways of defining physical sexual health; most of the available definitions focus solely on the reproductive functioning of the male boy or the sexual response mechanism. The importance of understanding the psychosocial contexts in which men live their sexual lives is at the centre of this book. To this end the definition of physical sexual health that will be applied in this chapter takes into account more than body processes and incorporates a degree of responsibility for both the self and others. Hendriks'[1] definition of sexual health includes aspects of this approach when he states that physical sexual health also incorporates the fulfilment of individual sexuality, enabling a person to share this with consenting others without jeopardising the health and well-being of other persons. This is the view of physical sexual health which underpins the issues discussed in this chapter.

Chapter 3 identified how the emergence of HIV/AIDS as a challenge to the health of people worldwide had a very positive impact in bringing the discussion of sexually transmitted infections (STIs) and sexual ill health in general into the public arena. Much has been written on the social, cultural, personal and even economic impact of HIV/AIDS, and there are many insightful articles and books on the subject.[2-4] However, the medical, social and historical legacy left by HIV activities in the years following the outbreak have also served in some degree to silence other aspects of sexual health. HIV/AIDS as a life-limiting, if not life-threatening, condition has a different contextual foundation than many other STIs and sexual health issues. This underpins the decision taken in this chapter to focus predominantly on 'non-HIV' aspects of sexual ill health, namely prostate and testicular cancer and common STIs.

PROSTATE CANCER

The incidence of prostate cancer

Worldwide prostate cancer is one of the most common cancers affecting males. In developed countries, it affects one in six men.[5] In the UK, it is the most common cancer in men, accounting for one in four of all new male cancers diagnosed, with a lifetime risk of being diagnosed as one in 13.[6,7]

Prostate cancer is an age-related disease and is uncommon in men under 50 years of age. After this the incidence and mortality rates increase exponentially.[5] There have been huge increases in the incidence of prostate cancer in the last 20 years. This is believed to be mainly due to the increased use of transurethral resections of the prostate for benign prostatic hyperplasia in the 1980s, where prostate cancer becomes an incidental finding in the tissue removed in around 10% of men, and the increased use of prostate-specific antigen (PSA) testing in the 1990s.[7] There are differences in incidence among different populations. Studies from the USA have shown as much as a 90-fold variation, with the highest reported rates among black African-Americans and the lowest rates among Chinese men.[8,9] In the UK it has been reported that men from the African-Caribbean community are three times more likely to have prostate cancer than Caucasian men.[10] However, there is some debate as to the cause of these findings. It is unclear whether this is cultural, genetic or familial. Where studies have been undertaken, it has shown that black men tend to present at a younger age than Caucasian men and that they present with higher-stage tumours, poorer performance status and a worse prognosis.[9]

However, it is important to remember that prostate cancer has a relatively long natural history and for this reason the majority of men are likely to die with prostate cancer than from it.[11,12] It accounts for 13% of male deaths in the UK, making it the second most common cause of cancer death in men after lung cancer.[7] Treatments have had a positive affect on the five-year survival rate, which has increased by 30%.[6,7]

Presenting with prostate cancer

It is not uncommon for men to present with advanced disease due to the late presentation of symptoms. This may be dependent on the stage of their cancer. Prostate cancer has four basic stages:

- Stage 1: The cancer is small and completely inside the prostate gland, which feels normal when a rectal examination is performed.
- Stage 2: The cancer is still inside the prostate gland, but is larger and a lump or hard area can be felt when a rectal examination is performed.
- Stage 3: The cancer has broken through the covering of the prostate and may have grown into the neck of the bladder or the seminal vesicle.
- Stage 4: The cancer has spread to another part of the body. In prostate cancer the spread tends to be to bones rather than any other organ.[13]

Lower urinary-tract symptoms such as poor urine stream, hesitancy, terminal dribbling, frequency and retention[14] are unlikely to be present in localised prostate cancer as they are more commonly associated with benign prostatic hyperplasia.[15]

There are three ways of detecting prostate cancer: PSA testing, digital rectal examination (DRE) and/or transrectal ultrasound-guided prostate biopsy.[15] There has been much discussion about the use of these methods and their appropriateness as screening tools. DRE has been commented on by some men as being an emasculating experience[16,17] which has prevented some coming forward for screening.[8] Transrectal ultrasound-guided prostate biopsy may also have similar connotations. This could never be used as a screening method alone as more men would have to be biopsied to detect just one with cancer.[18] However, the method that raises the most discussion is PSA screening. The aim of prostate cancer screening is to increase the chances of successful treatment by detecting cancer at an early, presymptomatic stage.[16]

PSA screening

Within the UK, PSA screening is not performed routinely. The main argument for this is that this type of screening does not meet the 10 principles which govern a national screening programme, as developed by Wilson and Jungner for the World Health Organization in 1968[19] (*see* Table 4.1).

PSA is found in blood and it exists in either complexed or free forms. Complexed PSA is bound to other proteins, whereas free PSA exists on its own. It is believed that men with prostate cancer will have a smaller proportion of free PSA and more

Table 4.1: Ten principles governing a national screening programme

1. The condition is an important health problem
2. Its natural history is well understood
3. It is recognisable at an early stage
4. Treatment is better at an early stage
5. A suitable test exists
6. An acceptable test exists
7. Adequate facilities exist to cope with abnormalities detected
8. Screening is done at repeated intervals when the onset is insidious
9. The chance of harm is less than the chance of benefit
10. The cost is balanced against benefit

complexed PSA than men with other benign prostatic disease. However, most PSA tests measure total PSA and free or complexed PSA testing is undertaken if the total PSA test is marginally raised, and not in cases where the total PSA test result is very high – suggestive of advanced prostate cancer.[19] This can lead to confusing results. PSA is found in men without prostate cancer and its value also rises with age in most men. A London study in 2005 detected cancer solely on the basis of a low free/total PSA value and found that using total PSA test results alone would have meant that most of the participants with cancer would have been missed by simply lowering the age-adjusted threshold for total PSA.[18] Up to 20% of all men with clinically significant prostate cancer will have a normal PSA result and therefore would not be identified through this test alone.[15]

However, what of the men themselves? How do they view PSA screening? An Australian study which utilised focus groups with 67 men – 34 who had been diagnosed with cancer and 33 who had not been screened – found that the men were unanimously in favour of prostate cancer screening. They believed that screening as a preventative measure was a procedure that every man was entitled to receive. Some of the participants likened it to cervical and breast cancer screening for women and felt that healthcare professionals have a responsibility to address screening with them.[16] In the UK, the Department of Health commissioned an information strategy for primary care for men asking for PSA testing. This includes an information booklet for practitioners, a factsheet on the PSA test for patients and a factsheet for staff.[15] As well as providing information on the test and interpreting the results, the booklet and factsheets also acknowledge that in order to have the test the man needs to be free from infection, have not ejaculated in the previous 48 hours and had no vigorous exercise during that time too.

Even though the UK does not have a screening programme for PSA testing, it does not mean that testing is not undertaken. The Second Survey of Prostate-Specific Antigen Services in England in January 2005 reported results from 118 laboratories, showing an increase in PSA tests of 39% in three years between 2000 and 2001 and 2003 and 2004.[19] PSA testing can be useful in monitoring the progression of cancer and the effectiveness of treatments. In an audit exploring whether DRE was essential for follow-up of prostate cancer patients, it was found that PSA was more reliable than DRE in influencing change in the management of these patients.[20]

Treating prostate cancer in the UK

Treatment options for prostate cancer depend on the stage of the cancer. In localised prostate cancer, the choices for treatment include active monitoring, surgery, hormonal therapies and radiotherapy; whereas treatment for more advanced disease concentrates on the latter three.[21] Active monitoring is a contentious issue for men, and it can seem strange that healthcare professionals are offering a period of monitoring without intervention. But men appear to fall into two camps on receiving a diagnosis of prostate cancer: those who wish to seek active treatment and those who wish to wait until further problems arise.[17] The benefit of active monitoring means that men are not having to cope with the potential effects of more aggressive treatments. Other factors that may influence men in their decision-making at this stage are age and general health. There is a general agreement that men with a less than 10-year life expectancy are unlikely to benefit from early detection because of the long natural history of untreated, localised prostate cancer and competing causes of death.[5]

Hormonal therapy can have a serious impact on the masculinity of the patient. The removal of a testis (orchidectomy) can influence a man's self-image and this may make him feel less manly than his counterparts. It is important that practitioners are able to recognise this and that support is offered. For some men, hormone therapy involves treatment with an anti-androgen or luteinising hormone-releasing hormone. Whilst these may appear more attractive to men, it is important that they understand the effects of these drugs. Some of the common side-effects of these treatments are hot flushes, increased body weight and risk of developing breasts,[14] all of which are attributed to being female. In addition, men may experience loss of libido and erectile dysfunction.[21]

Surgery for prostate cancer carries the same risks associated with any surgical procedure. However, the issue surrounding prostate surgery is that, though it may remove the cancer, it carries with it risk of incontinence and erectile dysfunction, which may not have been present at diagnosis. A study of 1,291 men revealed that only 32% of men had total urinary control and 44% were impotent two years after radical prostatectomy.[21] This needs to be explained to men to allow them to make informed judgements on their treatment options.[14]

Supporting men with prostate cancer

Providing support for men with prostate cancer can be challenging. Men appear to act in a variety of ways to gather their health information. The Internet can be useful, but men question the reliability of the information that they receive.[12,16] Family can provide an important role in assisting men with their decision-making around treatment options,[14] and some men will require information from professionals.[11,12] What appears to be necessary is that whoever is providing the support to men needs to listen to what the men really want from their support. Help is also available from charitable organisations. For example, Macmillan Cancer Relief has assisted professionals to establish a successful prostate cancer support group for men and their families in Chesterfield,[11] and The Prostate Cancer Charity has engaged with African-Caribbean communities to educate men on the function of the prostate, prostate cancer and PSA screening.[10]

TESTICULAR CANCER

The incidence of testicular cancer

Whilst prostate cancer is one of the most common cancers affecting all males, testicular cancer is the most common cancer experienced by men in the 20- to 44-year-old age group.[22] However, with only 2,000 cases diagnosed each year within the UK, testicular cancer is not a very common cancer. The incidence of testicular cancer has been increasing throughout the world. Within Europe, there is a clear north/south divide, with rates in Denmark being five times greater than those for Spain. The UK has rates that are above the average for the European Union. However, within the UK higher rates than average are reported in the southern regions;[23] but early diagnosis and improved treatments have contributed to a decrease in mortality and an increase in five-year survival rate.[22]

The reasons for an increasing incidence are unknown, but it is affected by risk factors associated with the disease. As well as age, cryptorchidism (undescended testis) is significant and increases the risk by 5–10 times.[22] A family history of testicular cancer, including previous treatment for testicular cancer, has been found to be significant, as well as the presence of HIV and having Klinefelter's syndrome, a sex chromosome disorder characterised by small testes and low levels of male hormone. Race and ethnicity are also important factors to be considered as the disease is most common in affluent Caucasians and rare in non-Caucasian populations, with the exception of New Zealand Maoris.[23]

Presenting with testicular cancer

The majority of testicular cancers are germ-cell tumours, which can be divided into seminomas and teratomas. Teratomas tend to occur earlier than seminomas, being more common in 20- to 35-year-olds, whereas seminomas are more common in 30- to 45-year-olds. Either type of tumour usually produces the same signs: a hard lump, swelling or enlargement, increased firmness, or pain and discomfort, either in the testis or the lower abdomen.

As with prostate cancer, a numbered staging system can be applied to identify the progress of the disease:

- Stage 1: The cancer is only in the testicle.
- Stage 2: Cancer cells have spread to the lymph nodes in the abdomen or pelvis. This stage can be further subdivided depending on the size of lymph nodes.
- Stage 3: Cancer cells have spread to the lymph nodes in the chest or above the collarbone.
- Stage 4: Cancer cells have spread to another body organ; for example, the lungs.[24]

The cure rates for testicular cancer are extremely good, with 98% being achieved in early-stage disease and 85% with more advanced disease, even to Stage 4.[25] The important issue appears to be the identification of testicular cancer as early as possible.

Nine out of 10 cancers are first found by the patient themselves,[22] as a routine screening programme is not recommended because of the comparative rarity of the disease and the high cure rates.[25] Self-examination of the testes for lumps and changes is recommended and should commence from puberty onwards, being undertaken on a monthly basis. However, most studies exploring self-examination of the testes show that it is poorly performed. In one London study, 49% of the participants had carried out self-examination in the past year, but of these only 22% had done so according to the recommendations of once per month.[26] The main arguments for poor adherence to self-examination recommendations may not necessarily be due to a lack of interest on the part of men. It appears that the lower prevalence of self-examination may reflect a more general deficit in health knowledge and perceived susceptibility.[27] Men report receiving written information on how to undertake self-examination, but they also report lack of knowledge and lack of confidence in performing the examination correctly.[22] This may explain why older men are more likely to undertake self-examination than their younger counterparts.[26]

Once a lump or symptom is identified, there can still be a delay in men seeking assistance. Over the last few years more has been understood about men and their health-seeking behaviours. However, relatively little is known about the illness behaviour of men with testicular cancer or their perceptions of why delays occur once they present with symptoms.[28] Where evidence has been collected, there are similarities in their findings. Men tend to fall into two camps: those who seek help quickly, within three months; and those who delay seeking help, three months and above.[28,29] Those men who seek help quickly tend to do so because they have a better knowledge of cancer in general, a better knowledge of testicular cancer in particular, a suspicion of a cancer diagnosis, or have seen media coverage of the issue in recent times.

However, the barriers to accessing help are many and reiterate the complexity of health and illness behaviours expressed by men. The impact of masculine self-image should not be underestimated. In a UK study, men reported fear of appearing weak, fear of loss of masculinity and fear of being seen as a hypochondriac as reasons for delaying seeking help. Also there was a concern about size of penis and having to show their penis to another man.[28] This was corroborated by an earlier Swedish study, which found that because of the site of the cancer some men felt unable to discuss their symptoms with anyone. However, this usually changed once a diagnosis was made and the men chose close family members for support. Even after diagnosis, a few men still felt unable to discuss their illness with anyone.[29]

Misinterpretation of symptoms has been identified as a barrier to seeking help for testicular changes. Pain appears to play a significant role in men seeking help. But it is not pain per se; the pain has to be at a level where it begins to disrupt day-to-day living.[29] Even when pain is present, some men will attempt to provide another reason for it; for example, a recent sporting injury or trauma to the groin, including recent surgery. Where pain is not present and the man feels fit in themselves, lumps are usually dismissed for the same reasons. Other barriers include fear of the examination being painful and how this may be seen in terms of their identity, and the suspected consequences of the treatment; in particular, sexual dysfunction.[28]

Treating testicular cancer in the UK

Treatment for testicular cancer will depend on the type of cancer identified. An orchidectomy (removal of testis) is usually undertaken, alongside radiotherapy and/or chemotherapy and surveillance. Seminomas are extremely sensitive to radiotherapy[25] and this may be all that is required for those men without metastatic disease.[23] For men with teratomas in the absence of metastatic disease, orchidectomy and surveillance may be enough. Men with metastatic testicular cancer should normally receive chemotherapy. Currently two or three cycles of bleomycin/etoposide/cisplatin (BEP) is recommended.[21]

Testicular cancer occurs when men are in their most sexually active phase of their lives. For many they have still to experience fatherhood. Treatment can affect sexual desire and function, although the problem appears to be more psychological than physical.[30] Therefore, prior to radiotherapy and chemotherapy, all men should be offered the option of sperm storage so that they may be given the chance of fatherhood at a later time.[21,31]

Another consideration in the treatment of men with testicular cancer is whether a prosthetic testis should be provided. It is recommended that this should be discussed with all men prior to their surgery.[21] However, in a large London study examining patient satisfaction following orchidectomy, only a third of participants had received a prosthesis, another third had declined, but the remaining third had not been offered the choice in the first instance.[32] Despite the fact that a third declined a prosthesis, 91% of the participants felt that it was extremely important to be offered the choice. Having the appearance of two testes was important to some of the men as this gave them the appearance of a 'normal' scrotum. In particular, 96% of those who were not offered prostheses identified this as being significant to them.[32] This is supported by a Dutch study where men without testicular prosthesis reported concerns about undressing in the presence of other males due to their scrotum appearing different.[30] However, it is also essential to acknowledge those men who declined a prosthesis when offered. The majority of these men were already in stable relationships and therefore it was not considered necessary by them and their partners to have a prosthesis implanted.[32] There is limited evidence that examines patient satisfaction following testicular implant after orchidectomy and this is an area where further research may assist men, and those supporting them professionally and personally, to make informed decisions.

Support and follow-up for men with testicular cancer

As the survival rate for testicular cancer is so good, surveillance for the future is required.[21] Survivors of testicular cancer have reported physical and psychological sequelae for many years after their treatment. In particular, the long-term effects of chemotherapy should be acknowledged. Physically these may include: vascular complications – for example, Raynaud phenomena being the most commonly reported;[31] nephrotoxicity, though findings are not clear; tinnitus and high-frequency hearing loss; and peripheral neuropathy.[33] Healthcare professionals who are aware of these issues can support the individual by monitoring modifiable risk factors such as tobacco use, hypertension, hyperlipidaemia and noise exposure.

Psychological sequelae are dependent on physical presentations. There is a wide discrepancy in reported problems, with some evidence suggesting less than 10% of testicular cancer survivors reporting psychosocial consequences[33] and other evidence reporting variations of between 25% and 75%.[31] However, this is not an area that has been studied well and this may account for the discrepancies, along with men's confidence in reporting psychosocial issues. Sexual function and fertility concerns are the most important predictors.[30,33] Therefore, it is not surprising to note that the most favourable outcomes of treatment include living with a partner, being fertile and feeling as attractive as before treatment commenced.[31]

SEXUALLY TRANSMITTED INFECTIONS

The incidence of STIs

STIs incorporate a wide range of conditions, including bacterial and viral infections which often present with few, if any, noticeable symptoms. STIs are possibly the most 'well known' and often misunderstood aspects of physical sexual health by the general population. Myths and legends associated with their mode of transmission, pattern of treatment and long-term consequences continue to affect people's willingness to seek help where an infection may be suspected. Psychosocial and historical issues concerning the stigma associated with HIV/AIDS transmission have added to the already complicated arena in which STI detection, monitoring and treatment takes place.

The 2005 surveillance report from the Health Protection Agency (HPA) gives a detailed overview of the current trends in STI infection in the UK.[34] The actual incidence and prevalence rates for the individual conditions shows some variation; however, the general picture in the UK is one in which there is a continued rise in the levels of newly diagnosed STIs and HIV infection across the population. This pattern is not unique to the UK, but repeated worldwide.[35] The key issue which unites the data from across the globe is the fact that sexual ill health, as illustrated through the incidence rates for STIs and HIV, are not equally distributed between males (or females) within any given population.

The general trend appears to be that of the burden of ill health being unequally borne by marginalised or socially excluded sections of the male population, including men who have sex with men (MSM), men from minority ethnic (predominantly black) communities and young men.[35] For example, in the UK young people are disproportionately likely to be diagnosed with chlamydia, gonorrhoea and genital warts. Men aged between 20 and 24 years accounted for the highest rates (56%) of the diagnosed cases of chlamydia in 2004.[34] In relation to HIV infection, transmission among MSM and heterosexual-acquired infection, particularly including individuals from sub-Saharan Africa, remain the dominant cause of new cases of male infection.[35]

The main message from the available data is that incidence rates of STIs and newly diagnosed HIV have increased over the past few years; however, in general STIs are easily treatable in most men. In addition, the wider availability and introduction of effective therapies for managing HIV have reduced the rate of AIDS diagnoses and deaths since the 1990s.[3]

STIs are usually transmitted as a result of unprotected vaginal, oral or anal sex or genital contact with an infected partner. Most testing for STIs in the UK occurs in genito-urinary medicine (GUM) clinics. These clinics have specialist facilities for testing and well-developed systems for offering the wider range of support services for coping with the psychosocial and personal aspects of being diagnosed with an STI, including contacting, testing and treating sexual partners. Contact details for GUM clinics can be found in the telephone book. Many GUM clinics are attached to main hospitals in major cities; however, contact details can also be obtained from local hospitals and community-based clinics. In the UK there is additional information available from the STI clinic directory on the website of the British Association for Sexual Health and HIV (http://www.bashh.org). An important aspect of GUM clinics is the confidential nature of their work. They will not inform general practitioners (GPs) of any results from tests or treatments, unless specifically requested to do so. This is an important issue for individuals who are concerned about the social stigma associated with a positive test result. Clients may attend one of these clinics at any age and be assured of confidential treatment (even if they are under the age of consent to sex, which is 16 in the UK).

As detailed in the introduction to this chapter, there are many publications detailing the treatment and management issues concerning people living with HIV. The historical and social contexts in which HIV/AIDS are experienced in society have a great impact on the management of the condition for individuals. This chapter aims to concentrate mainly on the most commonly treated STIs in the public health arena. Therefore, in considering the presentation, treatment and follow-up of common STIs in men, this section will focus on genital chlamydia, gonorrhoea, syphilis and genital warts.

Genital chlamydia

Genital chlamydia is a common bacterial infection caused by *Chlamydia trachomatis*. In 2004 it was the most common STI diagnosed at GUM clinics in the UK.[34] Genital chlamydia is asymptomatic in about 50% of men, which means that without a systematic screening programme a significant pool of untreated infection is likely to remain in any community.

Presenting with genital chlamydia

Due to the high rates of asymptomatic presentation in males, many men become aware of their possible infection risk through contact tracing of sexual partners. This is particularly true for heterosexual men, where routine screening for chlamydial infection alongside regular smear tests and other routine gynaecological examinations in women has been introduced in many areas over the last few years as part of the National Chlamydia Screening Programme.[36] Where men experience symptoms of genital chlamydia they often start between one and three weeks after becoming infected. Symptoms may include discharge from the penis, burning and itching in the genital area, and pain when passing urine. In some cases these symptoms are persistently present, but in others they may only last for a few days then disappear. Men with untreated chlamydial infection over a period of time may suffer from urethritis, epididymitis (pain and swelling around the testicles) or Reiter's syndrome, which is a type of arthritis associated with chlamydial infection.[37]

Testing for chlamydia used to rely on collection of swab samples from the individual. However, new laboratory tests have been introduced to diagnose genital chlamydial infections which are able to use noninvasive samples. In males this may be as simple as a urine sample. This has had a very positive impact on the uptake of screening, as well as working to dispel some of the fears around attending for screening and the possible procedures that an individual may need to undergo. The knock-on effects of these noninvasive procedures is that screening for chlamydia is now able to be offered in community-based or non-clinical settings. As a result, testing for STIs, including chlamydia, is now offered by some mobile health units, GPs, contraception clinics and young people's sexual health clinics.

It is recommended that where chlamydial infection is confirmed, the individual should also be offered screening for other STIs, which may be present without symptoms.[34]

Treating genital chlamydia

The main problems in chlamydial infection are detection and diagnosis due to the lack of observable symptoms in a high proportion of cases. Once diagnosed, chlamydial infection is relatively easy to treat and cure. Antibiotic therapy is the treatment of choice for chlamydial infection. A single dose of azithromycin or a seven-day course of doxycycline (twice daily) are currently the most commonly prescribed treatments used in the UK. As with many STIs, recurrence cannot be assured unless the sexual partner of the infected person also receives treatment. In addition, halting the spread of chlamydial infection in a population requires that all recent sexual partners (within three months preceding diagnosis) of an infected person should be tested and treated to prevent re-infection and further spread of disease. It is recommended that sexual partners of an infected person need to be tested whether or not they show symptoms of infection, and they may be offered treatment whether or not a positive diagnosis is made.

Systematic screening for chlamydia is a major requirement for controlling the spread of the disease. A plan to begin implementing a national screening programme for chlamydia was included in the Department of Health's National Strategy for Sexual Health and HIV in 2001.[38] The overall programme aim is to implement and monitor opportunistic screening for genital *Chlamydia trachomatis* infection for young women and men in selected programmes in England. Ten opportunistic screening programmes were implemented in 2002, with a further 16 programmes announced in January 2004. The aim is to have a full screening programme by 2007.[34]

Gonorrhoea

Gonorrhoea is the second most common bacterial STI in the UK. It is caused by the *Neisseria gonorrhoeae* bacteria. Recent trends show a decrease in the infection rates for gonorrhoea across the UK population as a whole since 2002. Infection rates for heterosexual men fell by 12% between 2003 and 2004, while a smaller decrease of 2.5% was seen among MSM.[34]

Presenting with gonorrhoea

Men are more likely to show signs of gonorrhoeal infection than women, who are often asymptomatic. In men, symptoms may include urethral discharge, or in the case of rectal infections they may experience discharge from the anus, anal discomfort and pain on anal intercourse. Gonorrhoea can usually be diagnosed by a swab taken from the penis. As with chlamydia, while most testing occurs in GUM clinics, some GPs, family planning clinics and young people's clinics now also offer testing.

Monitoring reports and public health research show that the rates of gonorrhoeal infection tend to be higher in inner-city, deprived areas and among many marginalised or socially excluded males such as MSM and some black and minority ethnic communities.[39,40] The population profile of urban and inner-city areas largely reflect the residential profile of these groups of males. Amongst these male social groups there is less likely to be easy access or effective uptake of care services, compounded by other determinants of ill health such as poverty, isolation and economic deprivation. It is therefore perhaps not surprising to find a higher incidence of STIs in these groups of males.

Treating gonorrhoea

The treatment of gonorrhoea is relatively simple in that, as a bacterial infection, it can usually be treated with an antibiotic (Ciprofloxin), often given as a single dose. However, in practice the effective treatment of this infection may be complicated by the fact that there are many strains of *Neisseria gonorrhoea* and some have developed a resistance to antimicrobial agents. This increases the risk of continued transmission of the disease and the chance of individuals developing adverse symptoms of continuous infection. This makes it important for anyone with suspected gonorrhoea to be properly investigated. As with chlamydia, all current and recent sexual partners of a person with gonorrhoea should be tested and treated to prevent re-infection and the further spread of disease. It is recommended that treatment should be offered whether or not they show any signs of infection.

Syphilis

Syphilis is an STI caused by a bacteria-like spirochete, *Treponema pallidum*. It is usually transmitted between partners during sexual intercourse. Until recently, syphilis was a relatively uncommon STI in the UK. A major decline in diagnoses of syphilis in males occurred in the early to mid-1980s alongside a similar fall in the cases of HIV transmission among MSM. This could possibly be viewed as a consequence of the emerging awareness of HIV and adoption of safer sex practices.[34] Diagnoses of syphilis in England in particular have increased substantially since 1997, driven in part by localised outbreaks in some cities such as Manchester, Nottingham and London. Records show that between 1998 and 2004 rates of diagnoses of infectious syphilis (primary and secondary) in males increased by 20%.[41] The pattern of spread of syphilis is unlike that of other bacterial STIs in that the largest pool of infection is not among teenagers; the highest rates are seen in older age groups, with the highest rates in males occurring in men aged 25–34 years, with a significant increase among MSM.[42]

Concern about the potential spread of syphilis amongst gay men and heterosexual men (and women) led to the development of new surveillance initiatives by the Centre for Disease Surveillance and Control (CDSC) in the UK. The new national surveillance system was established to improve insight into the geographic, demographic and risk-factor distribution of infectious syphilis.[43] The aim was to gather information to: (1) inform sexual health promotion interventions; (2) identify groups with significant levels of infection; and (3) provide data to inform understanding of the burden of syphilis infection.

Presenting with syphilis

One of the main problems with accurate diagnosis of syphilis is that the symptoms are not specific. At the outset the first signs of a primary infection may be the appearance of one or more painless but highly infectious sores appearing anywhere on the body (but usually at the site of infection). However, this is not always the case and the sores clear up on their own in 2–6 weeks. For this reason, many men may fail to attend for STI screening at an early stage as they may presume the 'problem' has been resolved with the disappearance of the sores. Left untreated, secondary symptoms may develop six weeks to six months after the onset of primary sores. These later symptoms are highly variable and may include the appearance of a rash on the palms of the hand or soles of the feet. Once again, the delay in development of these symptoms, the fact they may be located away from the penis or anal area and their non-specific nature, increases the likelihood of the individual failing to make the connection to an STI. Late syphilis occurs four or more years after an untreated primary infection. The latent (hidden) stage of syphilis begins when secondary symptoms disappear. Without treatment, the infected person will continue to have syphilis even though there are no signs or symptoms; infection remains in the body. Complications arising at this stage are much more systemic in nature, including damage to the brain, nerves, eyes, heart, blood vessels, liver, bones and joints. This internal damage may show up many years later. The signs and symptoms associated with the late stages of the disease include difficulty coordinating muscle movements, paralysis, numbness, gradual blindness and dementia.[42]

Syphilis is diagnosed either by detection of the organism in the ulcer when viewed under the microscope or alternatively the antibodies to syphilis can be detected in the blood. Once again, good practice recommends that a person with suspected syphilis should also be tested for other STIs which may be present without symptoms.

Treatment of syphilis

Syphilis is easy to cure in its early stages and a single injection of penicillin is usually sufficient to treat a person who has had syphilis for less than a year. However, all stages of syphilis can be treated with antibiotics, but additional doses are needed to treat someone who has had syphilis for more than a year. Alternative antibiotic therapy may be used for people who are allergic to penicillin. This treatment destroys the syphilis bacterium and prevents further damage, but it will not repair any damage to the body already caused by the presence of the infection.[44] It is therefore important that detection and treatment of the infection occurs as soon as possible after initial exposure.

Once syphilis infection is detected and treatment has commenced, it is recommended that the person must abstain from sexual contact with new partners until the syphilis sores are completely healed. The current and recent sexual partners of the persons with syphilis must be notified in order that they can also be tested and receive treatment if necessary. Treatment should ideally be offered whether or not they show any signs of infection.

Genital warts

Genital warts are caused by a virus, the human papillomavirus (HPV). More than 90 HPV types have been identified, around a third of which are sexually acquired and live predominantly in genital tissues. Genital warts are the most common viral STI diagnosed in GUM clinics in the UK.[34] This pattern is repeated elsewhere in the world; for example, the Centers for Disease Control and Prevention (CDC) in the USA report that more than half of sexually active men in the USA will have HPV at some time in their lives and about 1% of sexually active men in the USA have genital warts at any one time.[45]

Presenting with genital warts

Diagnosis is usually made by recognising the warts by their appearance or by looking for other evidence of HPV infection. Genital warts may not be easy to recognise as they could easily be mistaken for skin tags or normal skin; therefore, the person making the diagnosis should be experienced.

The majority of men who are infected with genital HPV do not have any symptoms. However, some types of HPV can cause genital warts which appear as single or multiple growths. They may be raised, flat, or cauliflower shaped. In men, genital warts may also appear around the anus or on the penis, scrotum (testicles), groin or thighs. Even men who have never had anal sex can get warts around the anus.[44] Warts may appear within weeks or months after sexual contact with an infected person or not at all. It is possible to have the type of HPV that causes genital warts, but never develop any warts. Certain types of HPV have been linked to cancer of the anus and penis in men.[24] However, as discussed earlier in this chapter, these particular cancers themselves are rare – especially in men with healthy immune systems. In addition it must be noted that the types of HPV that can cause genital warts are not the same as the types that can cause penile or anal cancer.

Treating genital warts

If left untreated the warts usually disappear, but this can take months or even years. Genital warts usually are treated according to their size and location. The most common treatment is based on the application to the wart of caustic agents or freezing with liquid nitrogen. A series of applications over a course of treatment is usually required to ensure the warts are completely removed. There is no immediate cure and this is often problematic for men who may find it difficult to continually return to the GUM clinic for treatment. The emotional burden of having an STI is compounded in the case of genital warts as even after treatment is completed warts often recur.

While most genital warts are treated in GUM clinics, some GPs, family planning clinics and young people's clinics now also offer treatment. This may help to reduce the personal and possibly economic problems associated with repeated return visits to the GUM clinic, which may be some distance from the client's home. Antibiotics cannot help as genital warts are caused by a virus.

Avoiding direct contact with the virus is the only way to prevent transmission and infection with the HPV causing genital warts. Sexually active men reduce their risk of infection by using condoms correctly and consistently during sexual intercourse. Condoms are the only form of contraceptive that offer some protection against sexually transmitted genital warts, but even then the protection is incomplete; therefore, reduction in the number of sexual partners may be advisable.

CONCLUSION

This chapter has outlined some of the diseases and conditions which impinge on men's physical sexual health. It has identified the importance of understanding men's physical health within the contexts of their lives. In discussing the incidence, presentation and treatment processes for male cancers and STIs, it reminds us to take into account other factors which may affect a man's ability to follow treatment recommendations or reduce their risk of contracting a disease. One of the important aspects of this chapter is that it has introduced the reader to the inequality inherent in the physical aspects of sexual health. It highlights that, even in relation to the small number of conditions discussed here, MSM, black and minority ethnic men, and men from other socially excluded groups bear the burden of sexual ill health. In order to fully understand and address the physical sexual health of men, we therefore require a broader understanding and appreciation of other aspects of men's lives in society. These issues and others are taken up elsewhere in this book, including psychosocial issues (Chapter 5) and the experiences of black and minority ethnic men (Chapter 7).

REFERENCES

1　Hendriks A. The political and legislative framework in which sexual health takes place. In: Curtis H, editor. *Promoting sexual health*. London: BMA Foundation for AIDS; 1992. pp. 155–166.

2　Holtzman D, Bland S, Lansky A and Mack K. HIV-related behaviours and perceptions among adults in 25 States: 1997 behavioural risk factor surveillance system. *Am J Public Health* 2001; **91**: 1882–1888.

3　Department of Health. *Effective commissioning of sexual health and HIV services*. London: DoH; 2003.

4　Pan American Health Organisation. *Understanding and responding to HIV/AIDS-related stigma and discrimination in the health sector*. Washington, USA: Pan American Health Organisation; 2003.

5　Remzi M, Waldert M and Djavan B. Prostate cancer in the ageing male. *J Men's Health Gender* 2004; **1**(1): 47–54.

6　Gavin A, McCarron P, Middleton R, Savage G, Catney D, O'Reilly D, *et al.* Evidence of prostate cancer screening in a UK region. *BJU Int* 2004; **93**: 730–734.

7　Cancer Research UK 2006. Prostate cancer. Retrieved 04/08/07 from http://info.cancerresearchuk.org/cancerstats/types/prostate

8　Bonhomme JJE. The health status of African-American men: improving our understanding of men's health challenges. *J Men's Health Gend* 2004; **1**(2–3): 142–146.

9　Heyns C, Lecuona A and Trollip G. Prostate cancer: prevalence and treatment in African Men. *J Mens Health Gend* 2005; **2**(4): 400–405.

10　Eaton L. Exploiting the domino effect. *MHF* 2006; **9**: 10–11.

11　James N, McPhail G, Eastwood J and James M. Establishing a prostate cancer support group. *Cancer Nurs Pract* 2005; **4**(1): 33–38.

12　Kelsey S. Dealing with uncertainty: caring for newly diagnosed prostate cancer patients. *Cancer Nurs Pract* 2003; **2**(10): 27–30.

13　Cancer Research UK 2005. Prostate cancer. Retrieved 17/07/07 from http://info.cancerresearchuk.org/cancerstats/types/prostate

14　Chapple A and Ziebland S. Prostate cancer: embodied experience and perceptions of masculinity. *Sociol Health Illn* 2002; **24**(6): 820–841.

15　Watson E, Jenkins L, Bukach C and Austoker J. *The PSA test and prostate cancer: information for primary care*. Sheffield: NHS Cancer Screening Programmes; 2002.

16　Ilic D, Risbridger G and Green S. The informed man: attitudes and information needs on prostate cancer screening. *J Mens Health Gend* 2005; **2**(4): 414–420.

17　Chapple A, Ziebland S, Herxheimer A, McPherson A, Shepperd S and Miller R. Is 'watchful waiting' a real choice for men with prostate cancer? A qualitative study. *BJU Int* 2002; **90**: 257–264.

18　Rowe E, Laniado M, Walker M and Patel A. Prostate cancer detection in men with a 'normal' total prostate specific antigen (PSA) level using percentage free PSA: a prospective screening study. *BJU Int* 2005; **95**: 1249–1252.

19　Department of Health 2005. National cancer screening programmes. Prostate cancer. Retrieved 11/07/07 from http://www.dh.gov.uk/en/policyandguidance/healthandsocialcaretopics/cancer/dh_4001754

20 Ragavan N, Sangar V, Gupta S, Herdmann J, Matanhelia S, Watson M, *et al.* Is DRE essential for the follow up of prostate cancer patients? A prospective audit of 194 patients. *BMC Urol* 2005; **5**: 1.

21 National Institute for Clinical Excellence. *Guidance on cancer services: improving outcomes in urological cancers – the manual.* London: National Institute for Clinical Excellence; 2002.

22 Rew L, McDougall G, Riesch L and Parker C. Development of the self-efficacy for testicular self-examination scale. *J Mens Health Gend* 2005; **2**(1): 59–63.

23 Cancer Research UK 2006. Testicular cancer. Retrieved 04/08/07 from http://info.cancerresearchuk.org/cancerstats/types/prostate

24 Cancer Research UK 2007. Testicular cancer. Retrieved 17/07/07 from http://info.cancerresearchuk.org/cancerstats/types/prostate

25 Grey A. Meeting the diverse needs of urological cancer patients. *Cancer Nurs Pract* 2004; **3**(1): 19–26.

26 Khadra A and Oakeshott P. Pilot study of testicular cancer awareness and testicular self-examination in men attending South London general practices. *Fam Pract* 2002; **19**(3): 294–296.

27 Evans R, Brotherstone H, Miles A and Wardle J. Gender differences in early detection of cancer. *J Mens Health Gend* 2005; **2**(2): 209–217.

28 Chapple A, Ziebland S and McPherson A. Qualitative study of men's perceptions of why treatment delays occur in the UK for those with testicular cancer. *Br J Gen Pract* 2004; **54**: 25–32.

29 Sandén I, Larsson U and Eriksson C. An interview study of men discovering testicular cancer. *Cancer Nurs* 2000; **23**(4): 304–309.

30 Incrocci L. Changes in sexual function after treatment of male cancer. *J Mens Health Gend* 2005; **2**(2): 236–243.

31 Rudberg L, Carlsson M, Nilsson S and Wikblad K. Self-perceived physical, psychologic, and general symptoms in survivors of testicular cancer 3 to 13 years after treatment. *Cancer Nurs* 2002; **25**(3): 187–195.

32 Adshead J, Khoubehi B, Wood J and Rustin G. Testicular implants and patient satisfaction: a questionnaire-based study of men after orchidectomy for testicular cancer. *BJU Int* 2001; **88**: 559–562.

33 Vaughn D, Gignac G and Meadows A. Long-term medical care of testicular cancer survivors. *Ann Internal Med* 2002; **136**(6): 463–470.

34 Health Protection Agency. *HIV and other sexually transmitted infections in the UK.* London: Health Protection Agency; 2005.

35 World Health Organization 2003. Sexual health. Retrieved 04/12/03 from http://www.who.int/reproductive-health/gender/sexualhealth.html

36 Adams E, LaMontagne D, Johnstone A, Pimenta J, Fenton K and Edmunda W. Modelling the healthcare costs of an opportunistic chlamydia screening programme. *Sex Transm Infect* 2004; **80**: 363–370.

37 Stamm W. *Chlamydia trachomatis* infections of the adult. In: Holmes KK, Mardh PA, *et al.*, editors. *Sexually transmitted diseases.* 3rd edition. New York: McGraw-Hill Health Professions Division; 1999. pp. 407–422.

38 Department of Health. *The national strategy for sexual health and HIV.* London: Department of Health; 2001.

39 Hughes G, Brady A, Catchpole M, Fenton K, Rogers P, Kinghorn G, *et al.* Characteristics of those who repeatedly acquire sexually transmitted infections: a retrospective cohort study of attendees at three urban sexually transmitted disease clinics in England. *Sex Transm Dis* 2001; **28**(7): 379–386.

40 Fenton K, Korovessis C, Johnson A, McCadden A, McManus S, Wellings K, *et al.* Sexual behaviour in Britain: Reported sexually transmitted infections and prevalent genital *Chlamydia trachomatis* infection. *Lancet* 2001; **358**(Dec): 1851–1854.

41 Simms I, Fenton K, Ashton M, Turner K, Crawley-Boevey E, Gorton RT, *et al.* The re-emergence of syphilis in the United Kingdom: the new epidemic phases. *Sex Transm Dis* 2005; **32**(4): 220–226.

42 Centres for Disease Control and Prevention. Increased transmission of syphilis in men who have sex with men reported from Brighton and Hove. *CDR Wkly* 2000; **10**: 177–180.

43 Fenton K, Nicoll A and Kinghorn G. Resurgence of syphilis in England: time for more radical and nationally coordinated approaches. *Sex Transm Infect* 2001; **77**: 309–310.

44 Holmes K, Sparling P, Mardh P, Lemon S, Stamm W, Piot P and Wasserheit J. *Sexually transmitted diseases*. 3rd edition. New York: McGraw-Hill; 1999.

45 Centers for Disease Control and Prevention. *Sexually transmitted diseases treatment guidelines 2002*. Atlanta, GA: CDCP; 2002. Report No. RR-6.

CHAPTER 5

Psychosexual aspects of men's health

Joy Hall

Key points

Across their adult years men can potentially encounter a diversity of difficulties affecting their sexual health and sexuality.

Erectile dysfunction is the most common sexual dysfunction experienced by men, with one global estimate predicting 322 million men affected by 2025.

Men require an open, genuine, therapeutic relationship with healthcare providers in order to address their concerns.

INTRODUCTION

The aim of this chapter is to explore the common problems related to sexuality and sexual health experienced by men during their adult years. Many of the problems encountered have serious consequences for the man's physical, mental and social well-being, reflected in their psychosocial and sexual morbidity. The chapter will therefore also discuss these effects, specifically focussing on the psychosexual consequences, together with a discussion of the role of psychosexual healthcare in the management of these difficulties.

The chapter begins with a discussion of the common sexual dysfunctions encountered by men, including their management, before moving on to the issue of male rape and sexual abuse. The chapter concludes with a review of the role of psychosexual healthcare.

DEFINITIONS AND PREVALENCE OF MALE SEXUAL DYSFUNCTION

Although several diagnostic approaches have been proposed to classify sexual dysfunctions, the most frequently used and widely adopted scheme is that contained in the *Diagnostic and Statistical Manual of Mental Disorders* (DSM IV). These categories (for men) are depicted in Table 5.1.

Table 5.1: Categories of male sexual dysfunctions

	Type of disorder	*Aetiology*
Desire	Hypoactive sexual desire disorder	Primary (has always
	Sexual aversion disorder	been present)
		Secondary
Arousal	Male erectile disorder (ED)	Global/generalised
		Situational
Orgasm	Inhibited male orgasm	Organic
	Premature ejaculation	Psychogenic
Pain	Dyspareunia	

In addition the DSM IV scheme also includes the sexual deviations, e.g. paraphilias. Paraphilias are disorders in which an individual experiences recurrent and intense sexual urges and fantasies involving either non-human objects, e.g. fetish, suffering or humiliation of oneself or partner (sadomasochism), or non-consenting partners, e.g. paedophilia, exhibitionism. However, other areas of sexual dysfunctions or sexual distress are not currently addressed by this diagnostic scheme, e.g. possible sexual addiction, hypersexual arousal disorder and sexual orientation issues. What is clear in clinical practice is that these 'clear-cut' categories do not truly reflect the complexity of the sexual problems individuals present. It is rarely possible to identify situations with a purely organic or purely psychogenic aetiology. In addition sexual dysfunctions are not all-or-nothing situations, but occur on a continuum in terms of both frequency and severity.

Co-morbidity of sexual dysfunctions is commonly encountered. Gregoire states that nearly half the men with low desire have another dysfunction, whilst 20% of men with erectile dysfunction (ED) have a corresponding low desire.[1] To add to the complexity of the situation, a number of interpersonal difficulties and issues also impact upon the individual. For example, the partner and the relationship have a profound effect on the situation. It was found that, for up to one-third of men with ED, their partner also had a sexual dysfunction; whilst Greenstein *et al.*[2] found the rate to be higher at 55%. The interplay between the various aspects of sexual difficulties experienced by a couple are frequently complex, circular and rarely have simple causal or consequential relationships. Indeed in clinical practice it is not uncommon to experience some difficulty in unravelling the nature of the problem, the practitioner often asking themselves 'Is this primarily a sexual or relationship difficulty?'

The exact prevalence of sexual dysfunction remains difficult to assess, with few general population studies. In the USA the National Health and Social Inefficiency monitoring found that 43% of women and 31% of men experience a sexual dysfunction at some time in their lives. Whilst in the UK, Wellings *et al.*[3] found similar findings. The prevalence rates for each of the male dysfunctions will be discussed separately later in the chapter. What remains clear, however, is that, despite recent advances in clinical research and perhaps a slightly more open approach to sexual dysfunction and sexual health, society still regards sexual adjustment and sexual health to be a luxury. It is suggested that the view of the UK government of sildenafil (Viagra) as a life-style drug to be prescribed selectively by clinicians under Schedule II (1998) bares witness to this. However, practitioners working in the field can testify to how much distress sexual dysfunction causes individuals and couples on a holistic level.

ERECTILE DYSFUNCTION

Of all the male sexual dysfunctions, perhaps the most well known, talked about and researched is ED. With the advent of easily available and user friendly oral treatments, ED appears to have lost its once greatly taboo status. Despite all the advances in treatment/management, what remains clear is the hugely distressing nature of this disorder for the individuals and couples experiencing problems. Additionally, despite the increased discussion about ED, few of the long-standing myths surrounding male sexuality have been banished. Indeed it appears in practice that the treatments themselves have produced myths of their own, with patients often having unrealistic expectations about the efficiency of medication. As practitioners it is essential that we provide accurate information (whilst not removing a sense of hope) and continue to demystify and challenge the old stereotypes and myths in order for patients to gain a clear understanding of their situation.

ED is defined as the persistent or recurrent inability to achieve and/or maintain an erection sufficient for satisfactory sexual activity.[4] As with the other dysfunctions, estimates of the prevalence of ED vary considerably, perhaps reflecting the fact that there are so many potential causes and that definitive epidemiology data is limited. The Massachusetts Male Ageing Study estimated that 5% of men over 40 years old, 10% of men in their 60s and 20% in their 70s will have ED. Individuals over 80 years old have an incidence of 30–50%;[5] whilst Pinnock *et al.* placed estimates of 2% in men under 40, rising to 86% in men of 80 years.[6] So what is clear from these estimates is that ED is an age-related but not age-dependent disorder. If one extrapolates from these figures, it is suggested that 20 million men in the USA may suffer from ED, with correspondingly similar numbers in Europe. Indeed Aytac *et al.*[7] demonstrated ED to be a globally experienced and growing problem. They estimated that, in 1995, 152 million men globally suffered with ED and they predicted this figure would increase to 322 million by 2025.

In order to understand the aetiology/causes and treatments of ED, it is necessary to have an understanding of the normal physiology of erection.

Physiology of erection

Penile erection and detumescence are essentially haemodynamic events, regulated by smooth muscle relaxation and vasoconstriction respectively. Erection occurs following a series of integrated vascular processes, resulting in the accumulation of blood under pressure and end-organ rigidity. This vasocongestive response is mediated via the autonomic nervous system. A pair of parasympathetic nerves from S2-S4 principally control erectile function, whilst sympathetic nerves from TII-L2 are primarily responsible for ejaculation and detumescence and are adrenergic responsive. The vascular processes of erection can be divided as shown in Table 5.2.

Table 5.2: Vascular processes of erection

Flaccidity	A state in which low flow of blood and low pressure exists in the penis. Sinusoidal smooth muscle is contracted and blood flows from the internal pudendal arteries via the cavernosal arteries and the helicine arteries to the lacunar spaces, and out through the open emissary veins (*see* Figure 5.1). Furthermore, the ischiocavernosus and bulbocavernosus muscles relax.

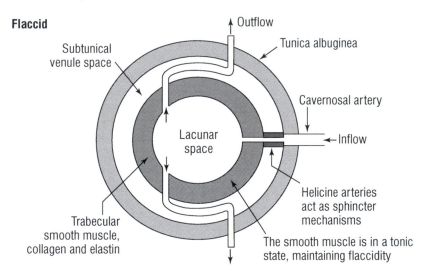

Figure 5.1: Blood flow and muscle activity in the flaccid penis.[8]

Filling phase	When the erection is initiated via any stimulus (physical or psychological) the parasympathetic nerves for S2-S4 provide excitory input to the penis, causing penile smooth muscle relaxation, enabling blood flow into the lacunar spaces.
Tumescence and full erection	The venous outflow is reduced by the compression of the subtunical venules and the emissary veins against the tunica albuginea, with a resulting increase in the intracavernous pressure.

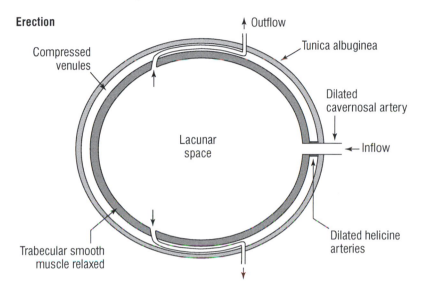

Figure 5.2: Blood flow and muscle activity during tumescence and full erection.[8]

Rigidity	The intracavernous pressure rises above the diastolic pressure and blood inflow occurs with the systolic phase of the pulse, enabling complete rigidity to occur (this also explains the pulsing or 'throbbing' described by patients – lacking in ED).
Detumescence	Caused by contraction of the smooth muscles of the penis and penile arteries, leading to a decrease in blood in the lacunar spaces, while the contraction of the smooth trabecular muscle leads to a collapse of the lacunar spaces and the penis returns to a flaccid state.

A number of chemical pathways (neurotransmitters) are involved in the erectile response. With the advent of oral treatments for ED, the practitioner must be aware of and be able to explain these to patients. The most important neurotransmitter appears to be nitric oxide (NO) induced cyclic GMP (cGMP), via the pathway identified in Figure 5.3.[4,9–12]

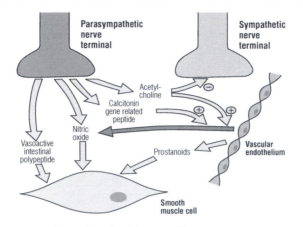

Figure 5.3: Neurotransmitters involved in erectile response.

NO is synthesised from intracellular L-arginine and released by the endothelial cells and nonadrenergic–noncholinergic neurones of the penis in response to sexual stimulation. NO then diffuses into the smooth muscle cells of the corpus cavernosa and activates guanylate cyclase, an enzyme which leads to the formation of cGMP then relaxes the smooth muscle of the corpora cavernosa by causing a decrease in intracellular calcium – erection then occurs.

Detumescence occurs when cGMP is broken down by the enzyme phosphodiesterase (PDE) type 5 (this is the enzyme which the majority of the current oral treatments for ED aim to target and inhibit).[4,12,13]

Causes of ED

As stated previously, sexual function (including erectile function) is a complex, multifaceted process, which requires co-ordination of psychological, hormonal, vascular and neurological factors. Alterations in any of these may result in sexual dysfunction/ED. Although it was originally believed that ED was largely due to psychogenic causes, due to advances in technology and medicine it is now recognised that organic causes are more common, particularly in older and middle-aged men. Although most causes will result from a mixture of organic and psychogenic elements, the balance between the two can vary considerably between individuals. Furthermore, whilst in cases where the cause is predominantly psychogenic, patients respond well to psychosexual therapy; in cases where the aetiology is largely organic, it may be unlikely that the patient will return to normal function without some sort of pharmacological or invasive interventions. It is essential that the practitioner identifies, through a thorough holistic assessment, the causes of the individual's ED in order that an appropriate treatment 'package' is arranged. This may well entail helping the patient and/or couple to adapt their sexual thoughts and behaviour to accommodate the use of medication or devices (*see* Table 5.3). In practice, this is often a hard task to achieve as so many people believe that sex is a 'natural act' that should not need any assistance, pharmacological or otherwise. The psychogenic causes of ED are outlined in Table 5.3. Each of these can generate inhibiting stimuli from the brain, which can block normal erectile function.

Table 5.3: The psychogenic causes of ED

Anxiety about sexual performance	Misconceptions or perceptions relating to sexual myths, lack of sex education/faulty cognitions
Anxiety about sexual identity/body-image issues	Relationship/intimacy problems
Anxiety or stress disorder due to work or financial-related matters	Sexual problems in the partner Life events such as concerns over ageing, depression, bereavement or other loss, surgery or chronic illness Psychosis
Psychological trauma or abuse Nature of sexual stimulus	Loss of partner attractiveness/habituation

Interestingly, although practitioners often associate anxiety with ED, it should be remembered it does not have a consistent effect on arousal. That is, anxiety reduces arousal in men with ED but increases arousal in those without. Performance anxiety is likely to have an adverse effect, whereas anxiety associated with novelty or threat is more likely to increase arousal.[1,14] Men with ED often hold 'faulty' thinking regarding their sexual ability and its linkage to the notion of 'real' manlihood. It has been shown that thoughts have profound effect on sexual response and modulate the effects of mood and anxiety.[14,15] It has been suggested that a man suffering from performance anxiety worries and anticipates negative consequences (when making love), thereby inadvertently removing himself emotionally from the pleasurable feelings associated with sexplay and intercourse. He participates by 'going through the motions', being unable to focus on his partner because he is totally and fearfully absorbed in himself as he performs.[14] This is a situation frequently encountered in clinical practice, where it is not uncommon to see couples where the initial performance anxiety has escalated into a general 'non-touch' relationship, with both partners being frightened of any sexual and non-sexual touching. It seems as though a huge wedge has been driven through the non-sexual intimacy and togetherness of the couple. It is essential that the practitioner recognises that multiplicity of interacting psychological factors effect the patient, while acknowledging that patterns of thinking arise from a complex variety of sources such as a person's/couple's cultural, religious, social, educational and family backgrounds, genetic factors and past life-experiences. All of these should form part of the assessment of ED and the other sexual dysfunctions discussed later in this chapter. It is also important that the practitioner remains open minded about these elements, not making assumptions about the patients' life experience – this is perhaps more of an issue for the inexperienced practitioner when they may be trying too hard to 'get it right' by ensuring every 'box is ticked' and applying knowledge in a more concrete manner.

Organic causes of ED

As with the causes of psychogenic ED, the organic causes are quite extensive. Figure 5.4 provides an overview.

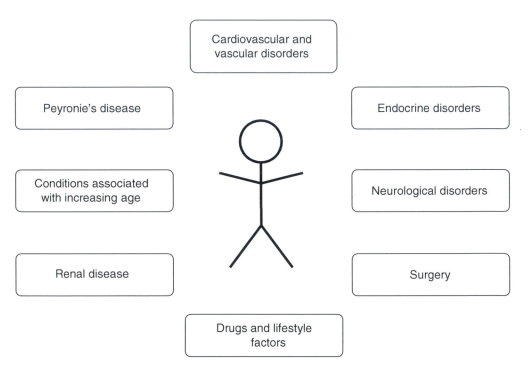

Figure 5.4: Organic causes of erectile dysfunction.

Cardiovascular and vascular disorders

Any disease process that interferes with the circulation of blood throughout the body will inevitably cause a reduction in the penile blood supply required for the maintenance of an erection. Indeed ED may be one of the first signs of cardiovascular disease in previously asymptomatic individuals. Atherosclerosis is the most common cause of vasculogenic ED.[16–18] There is extensive evidence that chronic cigarette smoking is a major risk factor for the development of vasculogenic ED because of its effects on the vascular endothelium and peripheral nerves. Furthermore, blood nicotine levels rise after smoking, causing increased sympathetic tone in the penis via nicotine-induced smooth muscle contraction.[19–21] Hypertension has also been shown to significantly correlate to ED. ED has been shown to occur in approximately 17% of men with untreated hypertension and 25% with treated hypertension.[22]

An additional vascogenic cause of ED has been shown to be hyperlipidaemia. It appears that this occurs as a result of impairment of endothelial-dependent relaxation in vascular beds (including those of the corpus cavernosa). Fortunately, these impairments have been shown to be reversible using lipid-reducing therapies and reduction in dietary lipids.[23]

As erectile function is also dependent on the veno-occulsive mechanism, conditions which cause failure of the mechanism will cause ED. Such conditions include: decreased nerve stimulation, decreased endothelial cell production of NO, extra venous drainage channels which may not be compressed by a compliant tunica due to collagen ageing, venous leakage, and replacement with connective tissue of the smooth muscle cells of the corpora cavernosa.[4]

Endocrine disorders

Diabetes mellitus is strongly associated with ED, ED being a complication which affects between 35 and 50% of diabetic men.[24] Diabetes can produce peripheral vascular damage and autonomic and peripheral neuropathy; thus leading to vascular and neurological dysfunction. Indeed, there is a close correlation between ED and other microvascular complications of diabetes such as retinopathy and nephropathy – so much so that it has been suggested that ED can be used as a surrogate marker for these other serious complications.[25] With Type 2 diabetes, ED may be the initial presenting symptom because the vascular and neurological damage has already occurred prior to diagnosis. For this reason, it is essential that the practitioner undertakes both a urinalysis (to detect glycosuria) and blood glucose test (to detect hyperglycaemia).

Less commonly ED can be caused by hyper/hypothyroidism, hyperprolactinaemia or hypogonadism (resulting in low testosterone levels and reduced or absent sexual desire – see the sections on disorders of desire for more detail).

Neurological disorders

Many neurological diseases can adversely affect erectile function. These include multiple sclerosis,[26] spinal cord injury or tumour,[27] stroke[28] and Parkinson's disease.[29] The effects of these may be as a direct consequence of neurological damage (such as demyelination) or indirectly, resulting from associated depression, relationship problems and anxiety leading to psychogenic ED.

Drugs and other lifestyle facts

Many prescriptions and recreational drugs are associated with ED (*see* Table 5.4).

Table 5.4: Medications associated with erectile dysfunction[4]

Psychotropic:	**Antihypertensives:**
Benzodiazepines	Diuretics (thiazides, spirinolactone)
Amphetamines	Vasodilators
Barbiturates	Sympatholytics (methyldopa, reserpine)
Opiates	Beta blockers (propranolol, atenolol)
	Ganglion blockers (guanethidine)
Tranquillisers:	
Phenothiazines	**Anticholinergics:**
Butyrophenones	Atropine
Thioxanthenes	Diphenhydramine
Antidepressants:	**Recreational agents:**
MAO (monoamine oxidase) inhibitors	Alcohol
Tricyclics	Marijuana
Serotonin re-uptake inhibitors	Nicotine
	Cocaine
Androgenic agents:	
LHRH (Luteinising hormone releasing hormone) agonists	**Others:**
	Clofibrate
Anti-androgens	Cimetidine
Oestrogen	Digoxin
	Indomethacin

It is true to say, however, that these drugs are often used to treat conditions which themselves can cause ED, e.g. antihypertensives, antidepressants and statins.

The effects of smoking have previously been discussed. It has also been shown that alcohol consumption increases the risk of ED. Polsky *et al.*[20] found that drinking between one and seven alcoholic drinks per week increased the risk two-fold; the greater the consumption the greater the risk. Therefore, it can be seen that advocating a more 'healthy' lifestyle – reducing or stopping smoking and alcohol, taking regular exercise, and eating a low-fat and low-salt diet – is an important part of the practitioner's role in both the prevention and management of ED.

Surgery and renal disease

Surgery to the pelvis or lower abdomen can lead to the inadvertent damage or destruction of nerves and blood vessels supplying the corpora cavernosa. The incidence of ED has been found to be particularly high in men who undergo urostomy, ileostomy or colostomy,[30] although surgeons are now much more likely to try to preserve these vital structures if at all possible. It is suggested that practitioners working with patients undergoing such surgery provide information about the possibility of ED pre-operatively. Together with facilitating discussions post-operatively, practitioners should make patients aware that it will take up to six months post-operatively for things 'to return to normal'; and therefore a true assessment of sexual functioning cannot really take place until that time. Radical prostatectomy and localised radiation has also been shown to cause ED.[31]

Men with chronic renal insufficiency disease are at increased risk of ED. This is true for men with chronic renal failure, often worsening if this requires dialysis.[32]

Conditions associated with ageing[33]
The effects of ill health and ageing on men's psychosexual health are those identified above plus (most commonly):

- Chronic obstructive airways disease
- Arthritis
- Alzheimer's disease
- Hypogonadism

Peyronie's disease and other structural abnormalities of the penis
Some injuries, surgeries, tumours and diseases of the penis can contribute to structural or circulatory problems that interfere with erection. In Peyronie's disease, plaques of fibrous tissue grow inside the dorsal portion of the penis, causing strictures, curvature of the penis and pain during erection. It is important that the practitioner asks the patient if they have noticed any curvature or alteration in the physical appearance of the penis.

Having a good understanding of the causes of ED allows the practitioner to understand the rationale underpinning the assessment process. It also allows them to offer good evidence-based explanations of the problem to the individual and/or couple concerned. Often, offering a clear explanation of the possible reasons for the problem is extremely therapeutic in itself, as individuals frequently have invented their own irrational explanations – which not infrequently lead to blaming and withdrawal behaviours, setting the scene for relationship distress. It is to the assessment of ED that our attention now turns; it should be remembered that, although the focus is on ED, many of the principles underpinning the assessment are also valid and valuable when assessing the other sexual dysfunctions discussed later in the chapter.

Assessment of ED
Determining the severity and possible causes of ED relies on careful and sensitive questioning. It is important that an accurate sexual and general medical history is obtained. There are pre-formatted questionnaires which can help guide

Table 5.5: Sexual Health Inventory for Men (patient version)

Each question has several possible responses. Circle the number of the response that best describes your own situation. Please be sure that you select one and only one response. Over the past six months:

1. How do you rate your confidence that you could get & keep an erection?
1   Very low
2   Low
3   Moderate
4   High
5   Very high

2. When you had erections with sexual stimulation, how often were your erections hard enough for penetration (entering your partner)?
0   No sexual activity
1   Almost never or never
2   A few times (much less than half the time)
3   Sometimes (about half the time)
4   Most times (much more than half the time)
5   Almost always or always

3. During sexual intercourse, how often were you able to maintain your erection after you had penetrated (entered) your partner?
0   Did not attempt intercourse
1   Almost never or never
2   A few times (much less than half the time)
3   Sometimes (about half the time)
4   Most times (much more than half the time)
5   Almost always or always

4. During sexual intercourse, how difficult was it to maintain your erection to completion of intercourse?
0   Did not attempt intercourse
1   Extremely difficult
2   Very difficult
3   Difficult
4   Slightly difficult
5   Not difficult

5. When you attempted sexual intercourse, how often was it satisfactory for you?
0   Did not attempt intercourse
1   Almost never or never
2   A few times (much less than half the time)
3   Sometimes (about half the time)
4   Most times (much more than half the time)
5   Almost always or always

SCORE

Add the numbers corresponding to questions 1–5. If your score is 21 or less, you may be showing signs of erectile dysfunction and may want to speak to your doctor or nurse.

the practitioner and patient through the process, e.g. the Sexual Health Inventory for Men (SHIM) (*see* Table 5.5). Questionnaires such as these may be used pre-appointment, and then used as a basis for discussion with the practitioner.

A crucial part of the assessment is the clarification of the onset and type of 'symptoms' the patient is experiencing. The main differential to ascertain is whether the ED is of sudden or gradual onset and present in all or specific situations, as this will help guide the practitioner to the potential aetiology of the problem.

The questions outlined below are taken from the NEED manual[13] and can help guide the practitioner to elicit the vital information about this problem:

- What is the problem with your erections?
  Useful cues:
  - Clarify the exact nature of the problem
  - Is it a problem only some or all of the time? (intermittent problem suggests psychogenic problem)
  - Presence or absence of early morning, nocturnal or spontaneous erections (in predominantly psychogenic ED, nocturnal and early morning erections are usually preserved; clarify the difference between ED and premature ejaculation)
  - Ability to achieve orgasm and ejaculation
  - How did the problem start?

- How long has there been a problem?
  Useful cues:
  - Sudden onset suggests a psychogenic problem
  - Gradual onset suggests an organic cause

- Do you regard your sex drive (libido) as being normal?
  Useful cues:
  - Compared to say five years ago?
  - Compared with your partner?
  - Compared with other men your age?

- What is your partner's attitude towards the problem?
  Useful cues:
  - Try to gain an insight into possible relationship problems
  - Try to establish if there is any underlying performance anxiety
  - Is the underlying performance anxiety a secondary effect of the problem?

- What do you think is causing your erections to fail? Have you and your partner done anything about it?

Useful cues:

  ○ The patient may be concerned about other health problems, such as cancer or diabetes that may need to be addressed

  ○ It is worth sharing views on possible iatrogenic factors and possible links to causation

  ○ It is useful to know whether the patient has already sought advice or obtained any treatment before consulting you

  • What are you and your partner hoping to gain from any treatments that might be available?
  Useful cues:

  ○ This is a chance to assess the patient's expectations from the treatments on offer

  ○ Agree realistic and achievable treatment goals for the patient and his partner

Table 5.6: Treatment for ED

Oral medication:	Psychosexual therapy
Sildenafil (Viagra)	
Tadalafil (Ciailis)	Vacuum constriction device
Vardenafil (Levitra)	
Apomorphine (Uprima)	Testosterone therapy (only if deficiency confirmed by laboratory tests)
Intracavenosal/Transurethral prostaglandins E1:	Surgery:
Cavaject	Penile prosthesis
MUSE	Ligation for venous incompetence

PREMATURE OR RAPID EJACULATION

Premature or rapid ejaculation (PE) is defined as the persistent or recurrent experience of ejaculation with minimal sexual stimulation before or shortly after penetration. Importantly it occurs before the man wants it to occur; according to Kaplan, an essential feature of PE is that the man lacks adequate voluntary ejaculatory control, with the result that he climaxes involuntarily before he wishes to.[48] Sometimes the situation is misperceived by the man as occurring too soon when, in reality, the ejaculation is occurring within what is considered an average length of time. The normal physical response is for the man to experience orgasm and thus ejaculate approximately 2–3 minutes after penetration. Indeed Kinsey, after looking at mammalian ejaculation and his interviews, postulated that, from an evolutionary perspective, such quick and intense ejaculatory response was probably adaptive – he found that 757 of his sample of 6,000 men ejaculated within two minutes of vaginal containment.[41] Whilst some others would suggest that sexual satisfaction of the female partner can be achieved by other, non-penetrative means,[42] it is important to consider how the difficulty is viewed by both the man and his partner. Although it is true that most women enjoy foreplay and direct stimulation, others believe that penetrative stimulation is better, or that sexual intercourse is the only 'real' form of sexual activity. Women who have these beliefs will be disappointed by and may subsequently lose interest in sexual contact – becoming rejecting of sexual intimacy with their 'dysfunctional' partner. Furthermore, men with PE are at risk of developing a general sense of inadequacy and failure, depression and other sexual dysfunctions, especially reduced sexual desire and ED. Furthermore, often there is a belief of sexual misinformation and myths about the 'staying power' of the man; sometimes coupled with comparison with previous partners' sexual 'performance'. Couples frequently do not understand the difficulty, with both partners making inappropriate inferences and judgements invariably leading to distress, and interpersonal and relationship difficulties.

Premature/rapid ejaculation is more common in younger men, suggesting that ejaculatory control is a learned response with greater control being developed through greater sexual experience. Furthermore, anxiety clearly plays a part in hastening ejaculation in some men.

The prevalence rates of PE/rapid ejaculation are difficult to ascertain. Frank *et al.*[34] and Nettelbladt and Uddenberg[35] reported 30% and 38%, respectively, in their general population studies. However, Catalan *et al.*[42] found 13% of their participants reported experiencing PE, whilst Simmons and Carey[36] reported rates of only 4–5%.

The practitioner should assess the patient's age, novelty of partner or situation, frequency of sexual activity (less frequent activity exacerbating the problem) and other factors that may affect the duration of sexual arousal. It is important to differentiate between ED and PE as sometimes the true problem is ED, necessitating prolonged stimulation in order to achieve an erection and therefore an apparently short period before ejaculation. They should also ascertain that the problem is not directly caused by substance use, e.g. medication or drug abuse, and that it causes marked distress or interpersonal problems.

Treatments for PE
A range of treatments could be utilised to treat PE. Some suggestions are:

- Condom use, e.g. Durex Performa (impregnated with a small amount of local anaesthetic)
- Simple measures – education, self-help books, local anaesthetic sprays
- Behavioural techniques – the 'stop and start' method, the 'squeeze' method, prolong ring system
- Pharmacological:

○ Selective serotonin reuptake inhibitors (SSRIs), e.g. Paroxetine 10–20 mg or Sertraline 50 mg daily or on a prn basis
○ Combination of the above with a phosphodiesterase inhibitor (PDEI), e.g. Viagra on a prn basis
- Counselling and psychotherapy – where pronounced psychological or interpersonal factors appear to be involved.

The practitioner should ensure the treatment proposed is individually tailored and culturally sensitive.

INHIBITED MALE ORGASM

Inhibited male orgasm refers to the persistent difficulty or inability to achieve orgasm despite the presence of adequate desire, arousal and stimulation. However, it most commonly refers to a situation in which a man is unable to ejaculate with his partner, being able to ejaculate during masturbation or sleep (nocturnal emissions).

Inhibited male orgasm is understood to be relatively rare and may be the dysfunction least frequently encountered in practice. Studies have demonstrated incidences of 3–10%,[36] with clinical studies showing incidences of 3–8% of men presenting for treatment, whilst community studies report incidences of 4–10%.[34,35]

It is important to differentiate inhibited male orgasm from retrograde ejaculation. Retrograde ejaculation occurs as the result of some medications, e.g. anticholinergic drugs, post-prostate surgery and occasionally as a consequence of diabetic neuropathy.[37] With retrograde ejaculation the man does ejaculate and experiences orgasm (although this may be associated with diminished pleasurable sensations). However, the ejaculate travels backwards, into the bladder rather than forward and out of the urethra. Possibly due, at least in part to its infrequent presentation, little systemic research has been reported on the aetiology of inhibited male orgasm. Table 5.7 outlines the identified psychological and organic causes.

Table 5.7: Organic and psychological causes of inhibited male orgasm

Organic	Psychological
Drug related:	Inadequate appropriate stimulation
Anticholinergic	Fear (of castration, pregnancy, commitment)
Antiadrenergic	Performance anxiety and spectatoring
Antihypertensive	Strict religious prescriptions
Psychoactive	Previous sexual trauma
	Hostility (towards oneself or partner)
	Difficulty 'letting go' and 'giving up control'
	Relationship disharmony
	Latent homosexuality

Psychological management revolves around reducing anxiety and increasing arousal, with sufficient, appropriate stimulation. Sometimes this requires the practitioner to 'give permission' to the clients to 'experiment' sexually, including using sex toys and vibrators, again demonstrating sensitivity and cultural awareness. However, if pronounced psychological or interpersonal factors appear to be involved, the practitioner is advised to refer the client on for more in-depth counseling or psychotherapy.

HYPOACTIVE SEXUAL DESIRE DISORDER

Hypoactive sexual desire disorder (HSDD) is notoriously difficult to define, evaluate and treat. It is associated with a wide variety of biological and psychological causes,[38] including stress and relationship problems, physical and psychiatric illnesses (especially depression), bereavement or other losses (including job), and medication (e.g. SSRI antidepressants). Rarely there are hormonal deficiencies/abnormalities (although clinically patients frequently perceive a lack of testosterone to be at the root of their difficulties, rarely wanting to 'easily' acknowledge the other, more likely aetiology, especially if it is lack of physical attraction for their partner).

DSM IV defines HSDD as 'the persistent or recurrent absence or deficit of sexual fantasies and desire for sexual activity'; again this is open to question, as the levels of sexual desire vary widely between individuals; therefore, the perceived 'deficit' may merely represent different expectations. Having said that, however, this mismatch of expectations can cause considerable distress for a couple and cause major conflict within the relationship. Individuals and couples frequently hold stereotyped and myth-ridden beliefs about sex and sexual desire, such as the myth that men are always motivated to be sexual (regardless of what else is happening in their lives); that desire must be present at the outset of a sexual encounter and does not/cannot develop gradually throughout; that arousal cannot take place without intense, overtly erotic feelings; and that feelings such as tenderness and warmth are not sexual.

Because of the difficulties with definition and diagnosis, it is difficult to gain accurate figures regarding its prevalence. Frank et al.'s[34] community study indicated a 16% prevalence, whilst clinical studies put the figure at 55% (for HSDD in both males and females), with men representing 60% of these individuals. However, Simmons and Carey,[36] in their review, give incidences of between 0 and 5%, whilst Meuleman and Van Lankveld[39] postulate it is in reality higher due to under-diagnosis.

Although hormonal abnormalities are a rare cause of HSDD, the practitioner must be aware of and test for the possibility of testosterone deficiency and prolactin-secreting tumours (e.g. pituitary adenomas, which according to Gregoire[1] may occur in as many as 10% of men presenting with HSDD). Should the man be hypogondic, testosterone therapy is now available in user-friendly systems, e.g.

transdermal patches and gels, not limited to the previous regimes of injectable esters. As with all the sexual dysfunctions and difficulties experienced by men, it is essential for the practitioner to undertake a thorough holistic assessment of the individual and couple presenting with HSDD in order to unravel what is usually a highly complex aetiology and to further offer a treatment 'package' which addresses this complexity. It would be totally inappropriate for the practitioner to focus exclusively on either the physical/organic elements or the psychological and social elements.

MALE RAPE AND SEXUAL ABUSE

Another important issue effecting a man's sexuality and sexual health is the effects of rape and/or sexual abuse. Whilst the 20 years up to 2007 have seen an increased acknowledgement of the effects of rape and sexual abuse on women, it is only relatively recently that the incidence of and effects on men have begun to receive the deserved attention. Coxell *et al.* found that 3% of men reported non-consensual sex as adults and 5% reported childhood sexual abuse.[45] One of the major problems faced by a male victim of rape or sexual abuse is the still overriding societal taboo on the issue, with many people still believing that male rape does not exist. Married to this is the belief that men are 'able to take care of themselves' and are supposed to be strong. These beliefs only heighten the victim's sense of confusion and self-doubt – with many ending up blaming themselves (for not being able to prevent it from happening).

The victims may experience a variety of effects of difficulties, including: feelings of isolation, depression, anger, anxiety, issues about sexuality and gender, substance abuse, self-harm, eating disorders, negative body image, fears about abusing, hyperconsciousness of body and appearance, and sometimes split or multiple personalities.

The most important thing any practitioner working with or encountering a man who is a victim of rape or sexual abuse can do is to believe what the man is telling them. In addition the practitioner must ensure the man feels psychologically and physically safe enough to disclose and discuss his situation (if he so wishes). Clearly, if the rape is an acute/current situation the practitioner must ensure that the man is advised about the legal and health screening which 'should' take place – as the man may be very wary of seeking legal recourse through fear of the police response. Many really useful publications are available for practitioners on this topic; these are included in the useful resource list at the end of the chapter.

What is obvious from the above discussions is that a man's sexuality and sexual health can be potentially compromised by any number of problems. So what then is the role of the healthcare professional in addressing these problems? In addition to those suggestions made in the section on the management of ED, the following section offers guidance to the professional.

THE ROLE OF PSYCHOSEXUAL HEALTHCARE IN MALE SEXUALITY AND SEXUAL HEALTH

It is obvious from the discussions throughout this chapter that a man's sexuality and sexual health is potentially altered or compromised by a multiplicity of factors. This area of practice poses a challenge to a lot of healthcare practitioners, as sexuality is regarded by many as a very sensitive and personal area of the patient's life, perhaps not to be intruded upon. And yet many patients look to the healthcare professional to give help, support and empowerment in this area. The degree of practitioner effectiveness will depend on their depth of knowledge and their degree of comfort in talking about sexuality issues. As a practitioner it is important to be aware that patients do not often voluntarily ask sex-related questions, possibly because of modesty or embarrassment. The practitioner therefore needs to create a comfortable, open, non-judgemental atmosphere of communication to facilitate the exchange of the patient's concerns. This can be achieved by ensuring privacy, patient confidentiality, appropriate timing and providing written/reading material specifically related to the patient's problem, together with the utilisation of existing counselling skills. It is essential to give the patient 'permission' to discuss his concerns by conveying that sexuality is a suitable topic for discussion. This could be achieved by normalising comments/questions, such as those adapted from Woods:[46]

> How, if at all, has your illness and/or treatment changed the way you feel about yourself as a man?
> How, if at all, has your illness and/or treatment altered your role as a man/partner/father etc?
> Other men who have had the same physical problem (illness/surgery etc) have told me that they have concerns about their sexual lives. Is this something you would like to discuss?
> If you could choose, what would you like to be different?

The answers to these questions help to determine baseline coping mechanisms, patient expectations and the learning needs of the patient and/or his significant others.

The practitioner needs to be aware that some men would find such a discussion unacceptable in their partners presence. Furthermore, for other men the discussion per se would be unacceptable, for personal, religious or cultural reasons. The practitioner therefore needs to be sensitive to these and other variables; they also need to acknowledge the patient's right not to discuss these areas of their lives.

A very useful counselling tool, which offers practitioners direction when dealing with patient's sexuality concerns, is the PLISSIT model:[47]

> Permission
> Limited Intervention
> Specific Suggestions
> Intensive Therapy

When adopting this framework, increasing knowledge and clinical skills are required as the intervention levels increase in complexity. However, using the four levels of involvement means that the practitioner engages in counselling at her/his own level of comfort and expertise. As the levels increase the practitioner continues to be free to make referrals at any time.

Permission

The practitioner can give the patient 'permission' to discuss concerns and problems. The willingness of the practitioner to discuss any area will help relieve anxiety and tension on the part of the patient. The practitioner can give 'professional permission' and reassurance that the patient's current sexual practices are appropriate and healthy. It is important, however, that activities that are potentially harmful to the individual or another are not condoned. Permission can also be given to experiment with new forms of sexual expression. It is important to recognise that permission can be given not to be sexual, if this is appropriate for the patient and his partner. Permission giving can be seen as preventative because it can resolve concerns that may otherwise grow into problems. This level of intervention is the least complex of the levels in the PLISSIT model and requires minimal preparation on the part of the practitioner. Furthermore, the simple reassurance that the behaviour is normal is often enough to alleviate the patient's concerns.

Limited information

Giving limited information provides patients with specific facts that are directly related to their areas of concern (having established these via the previous level of intervention). This information may relate to how their age, trauma, ill health and/or medical interventions affect their sexual abilities. Providing directly related information can be helpful in changing potentially negative thoughts and attitudes about particular aspects of sexuality, e.g. the de-masculinisation of ED.[49]

Furthermore, giving information that is of immediate relevance and limited scope can also effect behavioural change. As with permission giving, helping the patients to increase their knowledge about sexuality and answering questions about sexual concerns can be viewed as preventive, as these interventions can prevent or limit dysfunctional thoughts and behaviour.

The information may revolve around dispelling the myths that still abound in society in regard to sex, especially with respect to the 'real' man scenario discussed in the section on sexual dysfunction. A list of common sexual myths is given in Box 5.1.

Box 5.1: Common sexual myths and concerns

Myths regarding the characteristics of male and female sexual experiences and roles

Notions of what constitutes the body, e.g. 'normal' genital size, body shape and size, disability, etc.

Changes in body image or sexual functional ability; changes related to age, ill health or surgery

Myths about masturbation, oral-genital contact, sexual experimentation and fantasy

---

Providing limited information takes more time and requires more knowledge than permission giving, and frequently the two levels are used simultaneously. Patients are often concerned about what is 'normal' or acceptable behaviour, and are struggling to place sexual behaviour in the context of 'normality'. Therefore, there is the need for both permission giving and limit information to clarify misinformation, dispel myths or provide specific information. Information giving can be anticipatory or at the patient's direct request. Careful assessment of the need and readiness for learning, the nature and extent of the knowledge deficit and the most appropriate teaching method should be carried out before actual content is shared. Information giving is only helpful when the patient has a knowledge deficit. Here the practitioner's skills as a health educator are brought into play.

As stated earlier, in the section on sexual dysfunction, helping couples adapt to ageing, illness or surgery that can affect sexual functioning is an important preventive and therapeutic measure. For instance, consider a 60-year-old man who has ED following surgery for prostate cancer. Such a man and his partner would probably benefit from the following limited information-giving interventions: explaining to him and his partner the mechanisms of erection and how the surgery would have affected his erectile capacity; clarifying misinformation and dispelling myths that may contribute to negative feelings about this situation; discussing the treatment options available as appropriate; and discussing with him and his partner how these changes had changed/altered their own self-concepts.

Specific suggestions

This level of intervention involves directing efforts to assist the patient to change behaviour in order to attain stated goals by providing specific suggestions directly related to the particular problem. These involve direct problem-solving strategies or referrals for specific medical interventions; e.g. medication for ED or rapid ejaculation – for non-medical practitioners/nurses not working to patient-group directives. The suggestions made may help the patient to rethink the problem and make changes to alleviate the concern. Furthermore, the suggestions may involve giving practical advice, e.g. the use of lubrication (to aid penile insertion in ED), changing sexual positioning, or the use of condoms or the stop/start technique (in cases of rapid ejaculation). Fogel and Lauver suggest that in some situations giving a patient direct behavioural suggestions can help relieve a sexual problem.[50] They further state that this level of intervention is time- and problem-limited, with the nature of the problem treated at this level also being limited in scope. Problems of sudden onset and/or short duration are the most responsive to this form of brief treatment (perhaps one or two 30-min sessions). Sexual dysfunction that is generated by interpersonal conflict or of a long duration cannot be treated by this approach.

Intensive therapy

Here the concern may be a long-standing sexual problem that requires highly individualised therapy. This final level of intervention is the most complex and is used when the patient's problems have not been resolved after the three earlier levels and/or where the problems are ones in which personal and emotional difficulties are interfering with sexual expression. The therapeutic processes at this final level are longer and more involved and should only be undertaken by a suitably trained therapist. Poorman[40] suggests that healthcare practitioners should be able to work to level 3 of the PLISSIT model, but only within their own boundaries of comfort, knowledge and skills. The practitioners role in the provision of psychosexual healthcare includes education together with the use of counselling skills and techniques. The practitioner's abilities to develop an open, genuine therapeutic relationship with their patients will ultimately allow the patients the 'freedom' to discuss concerns related broadly to their sexuality. As stated earlier, a man's sexuality and sexual health are potentially altered or compromised by a broad range of factors. By adopting the framework proposed by Woods[46] – of assessing and addressing the man's concerns about their sexual self-concept, sexual role relationships and sexual function – the healthcare practitioner can guide discussion to cover all the bio-psychosocial elements of the men's life. In this way the practitioner can begin to give truly holistic care.

CONCLUSION

This chapter has demonstrated that men across their adult years can potentially encounter a diversity of difficulties which effect their sexuality and sexual health, especially their psychosexual health. Whilst focussing a lot on ED, the chapter has explored the ways in which the healthcare practitioner can help men and their partners overcome or adapt to these difficulties. The practitioner is in the ideal situation to address the issues early in the management of these men, before the problem becomes deeply embedded, empowering the men to 'take control' of the situation.

USEFUL RESOURCES AND ADDRESSES

British Association of Sexual and Relationship Therapy: PO Box 13686, London SW20 9ZH. Website: http://www.basrt.org.uk

Relate: Herbert Gray College, Little Church Street, Rugby CV21 3AP. Website: http://www.relate.org.uk

Survivors UK: Tel: 0845 122 1201 (Tuesday/Thursday 7–10 pm). Website: http://www.survivorsuk.org.uk

Useful survivors' book: Stott S (2001) *Out of the shadows. Help for men who have been sexually assaulted.* London: Russell House Publishing.

REFERENCES

1 Gregoire A. Assessing and managing male sexual problems. In: Tomlinson J, editor. *ABC of sexual health.* London: BMJ Books; 2001.
2 Greenstein A, Abramou L, Maltzkin H and Chen J. Sexual dysfunction in partners of men with erectile dysfunction. *J Impot Res* 2006; **18**: 44–46.
3 Wellings K, Nanchahal K, Macdowell W, McManus S, Rens B, Mercer C, *et al.* Sexual behaviour in Britain: early heterosexual experience. *Lancet* 2001; **358**(Dec): 1843–1850.
4 Carson CC. Male sexual dysfunction: diagnosis and treatment of erectile dysfunction. In: Kirby RS, Kirby MG and Farah RN, editors. *Men's health.* Oxford: Isis Medical Media; 1999.
5 Feldman HA, Goldstein I, Hatzichristou D, Krane R and McKinlay J. Impotence and its medical and psychosocial correlates: results of the Massachusetts Male Aging Study. *J Urol* 1994; **151**: 54–61.
6 Pinnock CB, Stapleton AMF and Marshall VR. Erectile dysfunction in the community: a prevalence study. *Med J Aust* 1999; **171**: 353–357.
7 Aytac IA, McKinlay JB and Krane RJ. The likely worldwide increase in erectile dysfunction between 1995–2025 and some policy consequences. *Br J Urol* 1999; **84**: 50–56.
8 Kirby RS, Kirby MG, Farah RN, editors. *Men's health.* Oxford: Isis Medical Media; 1999.
9 Anderson KE and Wagner GC. Physiology of penile erection. *Physiol Rev* 1995; **75**: 191–236.

10 Burnett AL. Nitric oxide in the penis: physiology and pathology. *J Urol* 1997; **157**: 320–324.

11 Saenz DE, Tejada L, Angulo J, Cellek S, Gonzalez-Cadavid N, Heaton J, *et al.* Pathophysiology of erectile dysfunction. *J Sex Med* 2005; **2**: 26–39.

12 Eardley I and Sethia K. *Erectile dysfunction: current investigations and management.* London: Mosby-Wolfe; 1998.

13 NEED. *Nurse education in erectile dysfunction.* London: Pfizer; 2000.

14 Weeks GR and Gambescia N. *Erectile dysfunction: integrating couple therapy, sex therapy and medical treatment.* New York: WW Norton & Company; 2000.

15 Cranston-Cuebas MA and Barlow DH. Cognitive and affective contributions to sexual functioning. *Annu Rev Sex Res* 1990; **1**: 119–161.

16 Montorsi P, Paola M, Galli S, Rotatori F, Briganti A, Salonia A, *et al.* The artery size hypothesis: a macrovascular link between erectile dysfunction and coronary artery disease. *Am J Cardiol* 2005; **96**: 14–23.

17 Ganz P. Erectile dysfunction: pathophysiologic mechanisms pointing to underlying cardiovascular disease. *Am J Cardiol* 2005; **96**: 8–12.

18 Billups KL. Erectile dysfunction as a marker for vascular disease. *Curr Urol Rep* 2005; **16**: 439–444.

19 Levine LA and Gerber GS. Acute vasospasm of penile arteries in response to cigarette smoking. *Urology* 1990; **36**: 99–100.

20 Polsky JY, Aronson KJ, Heaton JPW and Adams MA. Smoking and other lifestyle factors in relation to erectile dysfunction. *Br J Urol* 2005; **96**: 1355.

21 Shabsigh R, Fishman IJ and Schum CJKD. Cigarette smoking and other vascular risk factors in vasculogenic impotence. *Urology* 1991; **38**: 227–232.

22 Burchardt M, Burchardt T, Baer I, Kiss AJ, Pawar RV, Shabsigh A, *et al.* Hypertension is associated with severe erectile dysfunction. *J Urol* 2000; **164**: 1188–1191.

23 Leung WH, Lau CP and Wong CK. Beneficial effects of cholesterol lowering therapy on coronary endothelium dependent relaxation in hypercholesterolaemia patients. *Lancet* 1993; **341**: 1496–1500.

24 Enzin P, Mathieu C, Van der Bruel A, Vanderschueren D and Demyttenaere K. Prevalence and predictors of sexual dysfunction in patients with type 1 diabetes. *Diabetes* 2002; **26**: 409–414.

25 Ryder REJ, Hayward MWJ, Evans WD, Bowsher WG, Peters JR, Owens DR, *et al.* Detailed investigation of the cause of impotence in 20 diabetic men. *Practical Diabetes* 1993; **9**: 7–11.

26 McCabe MP, McDonald E, Deeks AA, Vowels LM and Cobain MJ. The impact of multiple sclerosis on sexuality and relationships. *J Sex Res* 1996; **33**: 241–248.

27 Ide M and Ogata H. Sexual activities and concerns in persons with spinal cord injuries. *Paraplegia* 1995; **33**: 334–337.

28 Angeleri F, Angeleri VA, Foschi N and Giaquinto SGN. The influence of depression, social activity and family stress on functional outcome after stroke. *Stroke* 1993; **24**: 1478–1483.

29 Brown RG, Jahanshahi M, Quinn N and Marsden CD. sexual function in patients with Parkinsons disease and their partners. *J Neurol Neurosurg Psychiatry* 1990; **53**: 480–486.

30 Petrelli NJ, Nagel S, Rodrigues-Bigas M and Piedmonte MLH. Morbidity and mortality following abdominal perineal resection for rectal adenocarcinoma. *Am Surgeon* 1993; **59**: 400–404.

31 Murphy GP, Mettlin C, Menck H, Winchester DP and Davidson AM. National patterns of prostate cancer treatment by radical prostatectomy: results of a survey by the American College of Surgeons Commission on cancer. *J Urol* 1994; **152**: 1817–1819.

32 Dailey DM. Understanding and affirming the sexual/relationship realities of end stage renal disease patients and their significant others. *Adv Renal Replacement Ther* 1998; **5**: 81–88.

33 Schiavi R. *Aging and male sexuality.* Cambridge: Cambridge University Press; 1999.

34 Frank E, Anderson C and Rubinstein C. Frequency of sexual dysfunction in normal couples. *N Engl J Med* 1978; **299**: 111–115.

35 Nettelbladt P and Uddenberg N. Sexual dysfunction and sexual satisfaction in 58 married Swedish men. *J Psychosom Med* 1979; **23**: 141–147.

36 Simmons JS and Carey M. Prevalence of sexual dysfunctions: results from a decade of research. *Archiv Sex Behav* 2001; **30**: 177–219.

37 Harland RHR. Sexual problems in diabetes and the role of psychological intervention. *J Sex Marital Ther* 1997; **12**: 147–157.

38 Rosen RC. Prevalence and risk factors of sexual dysfunction in men and women. *Curr Psychiatry Rep* 2000; **2**: 189–195.

39 Meuleman EJH and Van Lankveld JJPM. Hypoactive sexual desire disorder: an underestimated condition in men. *Br J Urol* 2005; **95**: 291–296.

40 Poorman SG, Smith JG and Robertson LL. Changes in sexuality related to physical and emotional illness and disability. In: Poorman SG, editor. *Human sexuality and the nursing process.* California: Appleton and Lange; 1988.

41 Kinsey AC, Pomeroy WB and Martin CE. *Sexual behaviour in the human male.* Philadelphia: Saunders; 1948.

42 Catalan J, Bradley M, Gallwey J and Hawton K. Sexual dysfunction and psychiatric morbidity in patients attending a clinic for sexually transmitted diseases. *Br J Psychiatry* 1981; **138**(Apr): 292–296.

43 Hawton K. *Sex therapy: a practical guide.* Oxford: Oxford Medical Publications; 1982.

44 Renshaw DC and Karstaedt A. Is there (sex) life after coronary bypass? *Com Ther* 1988; **14**(4): 61–66.

45 Coxell A, King M, Mezey G and Gordon D. Lifetime prevalence, characteristics, and associated problems of non-consensual sex in men: cross sectional survey. *BMJ* 1999; **318**: 846–850.

46 Woods NF. Towards a holistic perspective of human sexuality: alternatives in sexual health & nursing diagnosis. *Holist Nurs Pract* 1987; **1**(4): 1–11.

47 Annon JS. The PLISSIT model: a proposed conceptual scheme for the behavioural treatment of sexual problems. *J Sex Educ Ther* 1971; **2**: 1–15.

48 Kaplan HS. *How to overcome premature ejaculation.* New York: Brunner; 1989.

49 Caplan P, editor. *The cultural construction of sexuality.* London: Tavistock Publications; 1987.

50 Fogel L and Lauver D. *Sexual health promotion.* Philadelphia: WB Saunders; 1990.

CHAPTER 6

Sexual behaviour

John McLuskey

Key points

Men's sexual behaviour is usually described from a hegemonic masculinity viewpoint.

Men tend to view their sexual behaviour in terms of action rather than emotion.

Men will take risks in their sexual behaviour despite having the knowledge and ability to protect themselves.

INTRODUCTION

Most definitions of masculinity insist that to be a man you need to be having sex, of one kind or another. This chapter will provide a discussion relating to sexual behaviour in men. The complex realm of masculinity will be examined in terms of men as sexual beings and this will be explored to some extent within varying ages across the birth-to-old age continuum. In doing so it is hoped that common myths and stereotypes attributed to the sexual behaviour of men will be identified and possibly dispelled. The chapter will begin to raise questions about where men find their sexual opportunities and will consider their sexual risk-taking behaviour. In particular, the latter discussion will focus on condoms and their use to illustrate how some men perceive their sexual roles, rules and activities. This has been chosen as the focus for the remaining discussion, as the use of condoms in the prevention of unintended pregnancies and sexual ill health is a repeated health-promotion activity. The end of the chapter should encourage you to identify future opportunities for examining and addressing men's sexual behaviour in terms of identity, responsibility and expectations.

SEX AND MASCULINITY

Sexual behaviour in men tends to be viewed in terms of hegemonic masculinity traits. Sex is seen as being powerful, natural and driven.[1] Men are expected to report more frequent sexual activity[2] and this sex should be heterosexual.[3] It is uncontrollable, penis-centred, seeks to achieve orgasm whenever it can and relates to penetrative intercourse.[1,2] In summary, men are the assertors, the inserters and the predators.[1] However, this can be an often difficult and, for some, impossible set of rules to live up to, and it is important to remember that men's reactions and behaviours to sex are not in any way a single shared experience for men.

These beliefs about men and their sexual behaviour put men in an aggressive sexual stance and make women appear as passive, victim-like recipients. Whilst this may be more common in terms of sexual violence, for most men this is not the case and can lead to ineffective relationships with themselves and others, challenging their understanding of who they are and who they may aspire to be. Trying to follow the assumptions that men should initiate sexual activity, determine the form of such activity and decide when the activity should cease (usually after male orgasm) can lead to anxieties or withdrawal from sexual pleasure.[3] Some men who internalise the roles and values of masculinity may find themselves in a society where they are unable to cope, as the social norms for women have changed,[3] or they may feel excluded as they do not understand how else to function.

It is impossible to examine sexual behaviour in men unless there is some understanding of the way in which men might identify themselves as sexual beings. An easy way may be to consider the boundaries placed upon sexuality by society in that individuals should fit into the categories offered on many forms and documents: heterosexual, homosexual, bisexual, or other. But these boundaries do provide some understanding of how men might be perceived by those around them. The heterosexual chooses partners of the opposite (hetero) sex; the homosexual chooses partners of the same (homo) sex; and the bisexual may choose partners of either of the two (bi) sexes. However, these terms cannot be taken at face value when examining sexual behaviour. Self-identification by men can reveal discordance between their reported sexual identity and their actual sexual behaviour. For example, some men who have sex with men exclusively self-identify as heterosexual. In some cases these men are more likely than their gay-identified counterparts to belong to minority ethnic groups, be foreign born, have lower education and income levels and be married.[4] Their choice to self-identify as heterosexual may be influenced by religious, cultural or racial constraints, which define acceptable masculine roles and traits.

Despite the discordance reported above, there are other reasons why using sexual orientation as a defining factor in sexual identity alone is insufficient in understanding men and their sexual behaviour. All of the sexual orientations have further sub-divisions within them. Heterosexual men can be seen as being a stud, a real man, a mummy's boy, a new man, a married man, to name but a few stereotypes attributed to them.[5] Homosexual men have been stereotyped to be effeminate and therefore fall outside of masculine definitions. However, homosexual men have long used various descriptors to provide differences in their many sexual identities, such as the bear, the top, the bottom, the twink, the muscle man, the chub, the boy next door, and even straight-looking/straight-acting. In doing so they are able to demonstrate or reject traits of power, control and dominance.

SEXUAL BEHAVIOUR AND AGE

Age plays a significant role in the development of sexual behaviour in both males and females. From puberty onwards, boys tend to be more sexually motivated, whereas girls tend to seek emotional connections to sexual contacts.[6] Adolescent boys masturbate more frequently than girls, masturbate at a younger age and are more interested in casual sex.[6] Females are three times more likely than males to report being the less willing partner at first intercourse.[7] Young females are more likely to be vilified for their sexual activity than young males. Where a teenage mother may be criticised for allowing herself to get pregnant, the teenage father may be congratulated on his virility and 'sowing his oats'. Sexual promiscuity in young males is widely perceived to win respect from other males and this may continue throughout life.[3]

However, not all young males will approach their sexual experiences and developments in this stereotypically masculine manner, and this can have an important outcome on their sexual activity and health. In examining the reasons for using contraception at first sexual intercourse, it was found that young males who report feelings of love, fondness and intimacy as reasons for having sex were more likely to use a method of contraception at their sexual debut.[8] For the young male who is not heterosexual, other factors play a part in their decisions regarding sexual behaviour. These will be examined in more detail later in the chapter.

Another factor influencing the sexual behaviour of young males is where they receive their sexual education from. In the National Sexual Activity and Lifestyle study undertaken in 2000, young men reported their preference for sexual education in schools in providing them with the knowledge they required. Parents were seen to be a much lower and less useful resource.[7] However, this is in contrast to other researchers who have found that parental warmth and openness has a positive effect on the decision for contraception at first sexual intercourse, and that this had particular significance for young males.[8] As men age and leave educational environments, the focus of their sexual education and understanding becomes their friends.[7] Whilst friends can be a useful resource in supporting individuals through sexual experiences and relationships, their advice and knowledge may not prove the most effective when problems arise.

Little has been examined regarding the sexual behaviour of men after their teenage years unless they have experienced sexual ill health, such as sexually transmitted infections, HIV and erectile dysfunction, or unless their sexual activity is perceived to be deviant, incorporating fetishes or sexual offences. Studies may ask about numbers of sexual partners but rarely about healthy sexual decision-making. This is an area that still requires further examination and research.

The sexual behaviours and activities of the older male have begun to generate further investigations and studies. Previously these were undertaken to establish a biological understanding of the ageing process, but there has been a move to encompass the emotional and social aspects of understanding sexual relationships. The assumption that older people are asexual is no longer tenable and to perpetuate such misconceptions can only be considered ageist.[9] Studies undertaken in Germany, Australia and the UK all report continued sexual activity in over 50% of men above the age of 60 years.[9-11] However, there is a recognition that sexual practices have changed, one example being that the length of time from first thinking about intercourse to beginning intercourse had lengthened.[2] For those who are not sexually active, reasons given are loss of partner, general ill health, sexual ill health or sexual dysfunction.[10]

Comfort[12] is regularly quoted as stating:

> Old folks stop having sex for the same reasons they stop riding a bicycle: general infirmity, thinking it looks ridiculous, no bicycle.

Whilst he has been criticised for the simplistic manner in which he appears to disregard sexual behaviour in older people,[13] Comfort's comments can be seen to have some relevance in explaining the decline in sexual behaviour experienced by some older men. As we age there is a greater risk of experiencing illness, disease or infections leading to general infirmity. Even in the absence of disease and illness, natural ageing processes can limit mobility and function. Older men were once younger men and may have contributed to the various stereotypes regarding sexual activity in old age, usually that it should stop or become a process of ridicule. Therefore, it is not surprising that when they reach old age they are now victims of their own stereotypes. This can cause conflict for them in terms of their sexual feelings and their beliefs that sex in old age is not acceptable. Finally, 'no bicycle': Unfortunately ageing can also bring bereavement and loss and therefore some men lose their sexual partners. Commencing new sexual relationships in older age can be fraught with tensions and anxieties as it is for any age.[13]

The older male is changing and so is his environment. There is a longer life expectancy and with it an increased emphasis on quality of life, with individuals taking a more proactive attitude to their health, including their sexual health. There is greater access to sexual knowledge from a variety of sources and more liberal attitudes within the general population. Also there are new treatments for problems associated with erectile dysfunction. All of these together lead to a more educated and expectant older male, who is less likely than his previous counterparts to accept a poorer sex life as a natural outcome to growing older.

Traditionally relationships were formed when partners met through attending pubs, clubs, school, college and work. Sometimes the relationships were set up to allow one individual to be supported by another (double-dating) or were organised by friends who believed that they knew someone who would be a good match (blind dates). As newspapers and magazines became more available these started to include personal columns that allowed advertisements to be placed. Traditional ways of meeting sexual partners do continue for men, but there has also been an increase in the use of technologies. Internet chatrooms have become more popular, with electronic dating sites being developed for a variety of individuals with a variety of interests. These sites are popular among men as they allow them to develop an online discussion with a particular partner and set ground rules for the encounter prior to meeting, whether they are hoping for a lasting relationship or a one-off experience. For some men the use of Internet chatrooms allows them to undertake sexual activity from the safety of their own home. They are able to present themselves in a disguise that they feel will attract others to them. In many cases these men will develop usernames and nicknames that convey archetypal phallic size and power.[14]

Perhaps one aspect of sexual health that tells us a lot about men's sexual attitudes, values and behaviours is the way in which they use (or do not use) condoms. This will now be used to illustrate how some men perceive their sexual roles, rules and activities.

CONDOM USE

Condoms can provide an effective barrier to sexual infection and unintended pregnancy.[15] However, it is well documented that their use is erratic at best and non-existent at worst. There appears to be a greater use of condoms at first intercourse among younger males,[7] but there is also a reported increase in unprotected anal intercourse among heterosexual and homosexual partners in all ages.[16] Condom use among males can be difficult to measure quantitatively. Condom sales or a decrease in freely available condoms in pubs and clubs do not necessarily correlate with effective or appropriate condom use.[17] Therefore it is important to examine some of the issues affecting the decision-making of men when it comes to condom use. However, it should be noted that heterosexual males are often missed from research into condom use, as much of it has been influenced by HIV transmission among men who have sex with men.

The nature of the relationship between the sexual partners is an important aspect in determining effective condom use. Individuals appear to behave differently depending on whether their partner is a regular partner or a casual partner.

A regular partner can be described as someone who the male has developed an emotional partnership with or who is the main sexual partner for that male; and a casual partner can be described as someone who the male had sex with as a one-off encounter or has not developed an emotional partnership with. This differentiation is important as males appear to utilise different decision processes depending upon the sexual partner. With regular partners males tend to use emotion-based decision processes, whereas with casual partners information-based processes are more likely to be seen.[18]

There is more to consider than the type of decision-making process employed by the male. The importance placed upon the relationship also affects the decision to use condoms. Studies have shown that condom use diminishes in couples as the relationship progresses.[19,20] The reasons why condoms are not used with regular partners vary, but tend to relate to the emotional responses alluded to above. The abandonment of condoms in an evolving sexual relationship signals a growing degree of commitment.[19] This level of commitment is also seen by some men as an expression of trust in their partner and from their partner.[20] Some men would feel that by insisting that they use a condom with their regular partner would imply that they did not trust their partner to be faithful to the relationship, or to behave in a safe manner where that relationship allowed sex with others. Not using condoms can also be seen as a way of showing love and sharing intimacy.[21]

Trust relies on both partners accepting the unwritten 'rules' of the relationship, such as sex outside of the relationship (if sanctified) will always be safe. This has been described by some researchers as 'negotiated safety'.[18] Davidovich et al.[18] suggest that people in relationships should discuss negotiated safety agreements so that there are clear conditions to which partners agree to sexual contact outside of the regular relationship. If the agreements are broken further agreements should be developed so the relationship can still be maintained. However, this allows one or either partner to continue to expand the agreement within the relationship. In reality there are few individuals who have developed a clear set of agreements for sex outside of the regular relationship and usually this takes place without the consent or knowledge of the other partner. This has been seen in relation to men who pay for sex. In a Glaswegian study, one in ten men admitted to paying for sex, with around one in five of those reporting repeated episodes.[22] Of the one in ten men, 43% were in a relationship with a regular partner and more than half of these reported unprotected sex with both the prostitute and their regular partner. None of the men reported discussing their sexual activities outside of the relationship with their partners.

Another factor influencing whether condoms are used is the intention to use a condom in the first instance. Intention to use a condom tends to be associated with age. There is inconsistency in intention among adolescents, but this could be due to the inexperience of adolescents negotiating this behaviour. However, difficulties in negotiating condom use among casual partners can be seen in all age groups and not just adolescents.[23] Intention to use a condom is not necessarily linked to the actual behaviour. The response of the regular partner to condom use is an important factor also. Project SAFER (Study Assessing Factors for Effective Risk Reduction) was a longitudinal study undertaken in the USA with a variety of men in various sexual relationships, such as same sex, heterosexual regular partners, heterosexual casual partners and sex workers.[24,25] The study found that the regular partner's attitude and behavioural norm were influential in decisions concerning whether a condom was used for a variety of sexual practices. This was also affected by the perceived behavioural control of the men, which was established by whether they were the insertive or receptive partner in sexual activity. Insertive partners felt that they had a greater control of the decision-making process.

The relationship with casual partners could also be influenced by emotional responses, despite this being seen more clearly in regular partnerships. The male's view of his own sexual prowess could lead to him displaying a 'couldn't care less' or 'fatalistic' attitude to his sexual behaviour. This could also be seen in those men with a negative self-image or mood.[20] However, the lapse in condom use among casual partners could be attributed to many other factors, such as alcohol, drugs, distress, environment or opportunity.

Whilst the nature of the relationship has been seen to be important in suggesting some of the reasons why condoms may not be used, it is by no means the only issue. Since the early years of the HIV epidemic, it has been perceived that individuals could be encouraged to use condoms if they were educated about the risks of not using them. A study undertaken in 1998 reported that positive condom-use attitudes and high-risk knowledge were associated with high levels of condom use during sex.[26] Unfortunately the same study also found that continued risk behaviour was not associated with low-risk knowledge and poor condom attitudes. This suggests that knowledge does not necessitate appropriate changes to behaviour alone.

Rather worryingly a randomised controlled trial undertaken in 2001 appears to suggest that at times knowledge and education can increase risk behaviours.[27] This study randomised 343 gay men with an acute sexually transmitted infection into two groups. One group received the standard counselling procedure for an acute infection, whilst the other group received the same, as well as being invited to attend a cognitive behavioural therapy workshop. The workshop discussed negotiating safer sexual encounters. After 12 months follow-up, it was found that 31% of the intervention group had developed at least one new infection compared with only 21% of the control group. This was not the finding that was expected and it could be assumed that either the intervention was inappropriate or that it increased the confidence of the intervention group in being able to negotiate high-risk sexual situations.

Many men comment that unprotected sexual intercourse is a more pleasurable experience than sex using a condom. This has been described as the reinforcement value.[26] It is suggested that the subjective reinforcement value of unprotected sex could override the influence of attitudes, cognitions and skills in preventing ill health or pregnancy. For some men sexual adventurism and sensation seeking are major predictors of unprotected sex, which would support this suggestion.[19] Among men who have sex with men, this has been termed 'barebacking' – intentional unprotected anal sex with a non-primary partner. The pleasure experienced by these men may relate to the risk undertaken in assuming their sexual partner's health status, believing that they are HIV-negative, knowing that they are HIV-positive but that they are the insertive partner, or knowing that they are HIV-positive but that they are the receptive partner.[28] The challenge for individuals promoting condom use to these men would be to increase the desirability of using condoms. Strategies may need to more explicitly seek to lessen the reinforcement value of high-risk sexual practice and increase the perceived reinforcement value of condom use.

Perhaps the biggest lessons to be learnt regarding men's decision-making in using condoms for sex come from their views on conflicting advice and intuitiveness. Men appear to be confused by messages regarding safer sexual practices. A study undertaken in London questioned men who have sex with men to determine their beliefs about the accuracy of safer-sex guidelines.[29] The findings reported that the men perceived inconsistencies in the information they were given regarding certain sexual practices, especially in relation to oral sex. This has been supported by other studies.[20] The men in the London study felt that if they were having unprotected oral sex and it posed as high a risk as unprotected anal intercourse, then little is lost in moving from one to the other.

However, inaccurate risk perception is probably the most immediate barrier to effective condom use. Some men believe that they are able to intuitively guess whether their sexual partner has an infection.[19,20,30] This calculation tends to be made as much on the type of partner as the type of sexual behaviour. In this way men may seek sexual partners due to the way they look or the occupation they may hold, believing that they will be at less risk of any sexually transmitted infection. This appears to be despite having good knowledge of condom use and transmission of sexual infections.[21]

Unfortunately, men still require convincing that condoms can play a part in sexual behaviour. There may be an increase in condom use among young men at their first sexual encounter, but this use does not appear to continue for very long following this. Strategies need to be developed that will allow condoms to be seen as a part of the sexual act rather than an unwelcome add-on. Perhaps we need to think about addressing condoms in a more positive light rather than referring to them as providing a barrier, because men may see them not only as a barrier to infection and unintended pregnancy but also as a barrier to sexual enjoyment.

MOVING FORWARD

Sexual behaviour among men is a complex area that is still little understood despite advances being made among academic authors. Unfortunately, we are still some way off from understanding how men make their sexual decisions without exploring evidence relating to ill health or deviance. This chapter has tended to side with the common assumption of viewing men's sexual behaviour from a hegemonic masculinity viewpoint, and in doing so has omitted many other considerations. Men have been referred to and defined in terms of their sexual orientation but, as discussed, there are further subdivisions within these that warrant specific examination. There are also divisions within men themselves that warrant investigation, e.g. the influence of culture or ability, and this is beginning to be addressed, including within other chapters of this book.

REFERENCES

1 Plummer K. Male sexualities. In: Kimmel MS, Hearn J and Connell RW, editors. *Handbook of studies on men & masculinities.* Thousand Oaks, CA: Sage Publications; 2005.

2 Eardley I, Dean J, Barnes T, Kirby M, Glasser D and Solanki J. The sexual habits of British men and women over 40 years old. *BJU Int* 2004; **93**: 563–567.

3 Lee C and Owens G. *The psychology of men's health.* Buckingham: Open University Press; 2002.

4 Pathela P, Hajat A, Schillinger J, Blank S, Sell R and Mostashari F. Discordance between sexual behaviour and self-reported sexual identity: a population-based survey of New York City men. *Ann Intern Med* 2006; **145**: 416–425.

5 Van Ooijen E and Charnock A. *Sexuality and patient care: a guide for nurses and teachers.* London: Chapman and Hall; 1994.

6 Hiller J. Gender differences in sexual motivation. *J Men Health Gend* 2005; **2**(3): 339–345.

7 Wellings K, Nanchahal K, Macdowell W, McManus S, Rens B, Mercer C, *et al.* Sexual behaviour in Britain: early heterosexual experience. *Lancet* 2001; **358**(Dec): 1843–1850.

8 Stone N and Ingram R. Factors affecting British teenagers' contraceptive use at first intercourse: the importance of partner communication. *Perspect Sex Reprod Health* 2002; **34**(4): 191–197.

9 Minichiello V, Plummer D and Loxton D. Factors predicting sexual relationships in older people: an Australian study. *Aust J Ageing* 2004; **23**(3): 125–130.

10 Beutel M, Schumacher J, Weidner W and Brahler E. Sexual activity, sexual and partnership satisfaction in ageing men – results from a German representative community study. *Andrologia* 2002; **34**: 22–28.

11 Edley N and Wetherall M. *Men in perspective: practice, power and identity.* Hemel Hempstead: Harvester Wheatsheaf; 1995.

12 Comfort A. Sexuality in old age. *J Am Geriatr Soc* 1974; **22**(10): 440–442.

13 Wallace M. Sexuality and aging in long-term care. *Ann Long Term Care* 2003; **11**(2): 53–59.

14 McKay J, Mikosza J and Hutchins B. 'Gentlemen, the lunchbox has landed': representations of masculinities and men's bodies in the popular media. In: Kimmel MS, Hearn J and Connell RW, editors. *Handbook of studies on men & masculinities*. Thousand Oaks, CA: Sage Publications; 2005.

15 Slaymaker E. A critique of international indicators of sexual risk behaviours. *Sex Transm Infect* 2004; **80**(11 Suppl): 13–21.

16 Johnson A, Mercer CH, Erens B, Copas AJ, McManus S, Wellings K, *et al.* Sexual behaviour in Britain: partnerships, practices and HIV risk behaviours. *Lancet* 2001; **358**: 1835–1842.

17 Meekers D and van Rossem R. Explaining inconsistencies between data on condom use and condom sales. *BMC Health Serv Res* 2005; **5**: 5.

18 Davidovich U, Wit JBF de and Stroebe W. Assessing sexual risk behaviour of young gay men in primary relationships: the incorporation of negotiated safety and negotiated safety compliance. *AIDS* 2000; **14**(6): 701–706.

19 Donovan B and Ross MW. Preventing HIV: determinants of sexual behaviour. *Lancet* 2000; **355**: 1897–1901.

20 Adam B, Sears A and Schellenberg EG. Accounting for unsafe sex: interviews with men who have sex with men. *J Sex Res* 2000; **37**(1): 24–36.

21 Fenton K and Power R. Why do homosexual men continue to practise unsafe sex? A critical review of a qualitative research paper. *Genitourin Med* 1997; **73**: 404–409.

22 Groom T and Nandwani R. Characteristics of men who pay for sex: a UK sexual health clinic survey. *Sex Transm Infect* 2006; **82**: 364–367.

23 Sheeran P and Orbell S. Do intentions predict condom use? Meta-analysis and examination of six moderator variables. *Br J Soc Psychol* 1998; **37**: 231–250.

24 Levina M, Dantas G, Fishbein M, von Haeften I and Montano D. Factors influencing MSM's intentions to always use condoms for vaginal, anal and oral sex with their regular partners. *Psychol Health Med* 2001; **6**(2): 191–205.

25 Montano D, Kasprzyk D, von Haeften I and Fishbein M. Toward an understanding of condom use behaviours: a theoretical and methodological overview of Project SAFER. *Psychol Health Med* 2001; **6**(2): 139–149.

26 Kelly J and Kalichman SC. Reinforcement value in unsafe sex as a predictor of condom use and continued HIV/AIDS risk behaviour among gay and bisexual men. *Health Psychol* 1998; **17**(4): 328–335.

27 Imrie J, Stephenson JM, Cowan FM, Wanigaratne S, Billington AJP, Copas AJ, *et al.* A cognitive behavioural intervention to reduce sexually transmitted infections among gay men: randomised trial. *BMJ* 2001; **322**: 1451–1456.

28 Mansergh G, Marks G, Colfax GN, Guzman R, Rader M and Buchbinder S. 'Barebacking' in a diverse sample of men who have sex with men. *AIDS* 2002; **16**: 653–659.

29 Phillips KD, Sowell RL and Misener TR. Relationships among HIV risk beliefs, attitudes and behaviours in sexually active seronegative gay men. *Nurs Connect* 1998; **11**(1): 5–24.

30 Dodds J, Nardone A, Mercey DE and Johnson AM. Increase in high risk sexual behaviour among homosexual men, London 1996–8: a cross sectional questionnaire study. *BMJ* 2000; **320**: 1510–1511.

CHAPTER 7

Sexual health promotion for black and minority ethnic men

Vanessa McFarlane and Laura Serrant-Green

Key points

Black and minority ethnic men are shown to be at disproportionately higher risk of sexual ill health.

Addressing the sexual health needs of black and minority ethnic men requires a contextualised approach which includes recognition of diversity and difference of experience.

Community-based initiatives which involve local stakeholders and community organisations provide a positive example for developing an integrated approach to sexual health.

INTRODUCTION

Ethnicity has a major impact on our lives. Your ethnicity defines who you are. It tells your history, it's something you can be proud of; but it may also be something that limits you, fits you into boxes, can feel like a burden or be used by others to make assumptions about you.

Studies reveal that the impact of ethnicity stretches beyond mere identity to influence whether we achieve educationally,[1] have a higher risk of being involved in criminal activity,[2] live in certain areas and ultimately our health and life expectancy.[3]

This chapter aims to consider the key issues impacting on the sexual health of men from black and minority ethnic (BME) communities. The discussion will be framed around consideration of the following issues:

- What influences the sexual health of BME men?
- Why does there appear to be disproportionately much higher levels of sexual ill health in some groups of BME men than the general population?

The chapter also uses case study presentations of a variety of community-based schemes in the Midlands, UK, to demonstrate examples of good practice in sexual health promotion with BME men. The chapter concludes by looking at possible ways forward in maximising the health and ultimately life chances of this section of the population.

DEFINING BME

In today's society, identity matters. The possible variations in experiences arising out of the interplay between gender, races and ethnicities in society mean it is important that any discussion of identity related to race and/or ethnicity clarifies the frame of reference used in the discussion. To this end this first section concludes by identifying how the terms 'black' and 'minority ethnic' are used throughout this chapter.

USE OF THE TERM 'BLACK'

The term 'black' is used in this study as a political term to identify peoples of African, African-Caribbean and South Asian origin. It is a term increasingly accepted by the members of the groups themselves as representing a unity of experience of racism, discrimination and prejudice amongst people whose skin colour is not white. Utilising this definition in no way infers a belief in a homogeneous black identity, but acknowledges the modifying effects of other socially determined factors such as gender, education and class on experiences. We therefore present this chapter while embracing the diversity of black experience within and between black individuals and communities.

USE OF THE TERM 'MINORITY ETHNIC'

There exists within Britain, as in other parts of the world, a host of communities who by virtue of a difference in language, customs, country of origin, religion, norms and values are different from the majority ethnic populations. These communities, like black communities, are recognised as having minority ethnic identities, may also be white or do not define themselves as black. In relation to health-needs assessment, service planning and social provision, however, they also experience a degree of discrimination that is often hidden. These are the minority ethnic communities referred to in this study.

The most important aspect of any 'definition' of ethnic identity is accepting that individuals and groups 'self-assign' their identities. These often exist in contrast or conflict with the socially determined categorisations of wider society. Managing and living with these contradictions between personal and external expectations are an integral part of the lives of many BME communities. The consequences of living with these tensions may be reflected in the available choices and decisions they make about their (sexual) health. In this chapter the focus will primarily be on the experiences of black African, black Caribbean and Asian men who comprise the largest proportion of BME males in Britain.[4]

INEQUALITIES IN HEALTH

There is a generally held belief that belonging to a BME group is bad for your health. Reports demonstrate that BME communities experience disproportionately higher rates of chronic illnesses such as diabetes,[5] are more likely to be diagnosed with a mental health problem[6] and are likely to report experiencing poor healthcare.[7,8] Blind acceptance of this data as indicative of some inherent aspects of BME individuals, however, is recognised as being folly. Critical review of the research reports reveals that an inevitable correlation between belonging to a BME community and poor health is not the case. There are many factors that have to be added into the equation which impact on health and illness, such as socio-economic group, inequality and racism within provision or access to services, as well as genetic inheritance of certain life-limiting illnesses. A large proportion of BME groups belong to lower socio-economic classes and research has told us for many years that this has a direct affect on health. There is evidence, for example, that Bangladeshis, Pakistanis and Caribbeans in Western society are overall at risk of poorer health than whites in many countries.[9,10]

SEXUAL HEALTH

The politically and socially sensitive nature of the subjects of ethnicity and sexual health lie at the heart of investigation into black Caribbean men and their sexual health. These issues have historically influenced the types of British-based research that have been conducted in these areas and the willingness of researchers to select these as subjects of study. Attempts to conduct a national survey on sexual attitudes and lifestyles in Britain in the early 1980s, for example, were blocked by the government of the time as this was deemed inappropriate use of public funds and politically problematic.[11] Research and statistics on the sexual health of BME communities in Britain is still in the early stages. There are quite a few studies of

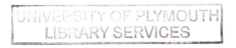

African communities and HIV, but much less around generic sexual health and other BME groups. What has been done seems to be in small pockets in and around London rather than more national studies. However, we do know that the UK's BME populations continue to be disproportionately affected by poor sexual health. The groups affected and their experiences of HIV and sexually transmitted infections (STIs) vary greatly.[12–14]

BME groups are diverse within themselves and in their pattern of distribution across the UK. For example, many cities in the Midlands have an established Caribbean community that has had a presence since the late 1940s to 1950s, when people came to the UK for economic reasons. These established communities have been joined in recent years by a largely new and growing African community, which includes refugees and asylum seekers as well as economic migrants and students. These two groups are a good example of how, even within the same ethnic groups, people will identify themselves as separate and distinct from each other. The nature and pattern of migration combined with the differing cultural experiences of the people in these communities suggests they will have different needs in relation to their sexual health. This is also the case within Asian communities in the Midlands, where there is a predominant Pakistani Muslim community, with smaller Indian Sikh and Hindu communities – most of these communities came as economic migrants in the 1950s, but have also been joined by Pakistani refugee and asylum seekers.

Views about sexual health will vary among these communities, although there is a general consensus amongst these groups that sex outside of marriage is viewed as wrong and discussions about sex are taboo. Health service providers and nurse researchers have been accused of being particularly reluctant in adopting a critical approach to the needs of BME clients, particularly in acknowledging the effects of race and racism on the health and life chances of BME populations.[15–17] As a result the wider health implications resulting from the interplay of ethnicity, class or gender on sexual health have received little attention.

Dr Nicola Low[18] carried out research on the sexual health of BME groups in the late 1990s and noted that differences between black ethnic groups are not well appreciated as they become lumped together. Against this backdrop it is perhaps pertinent to consider how the sexual health of BME communities is affected.

The Trust for the Study of Adolescence for Naz Project London[35] found that teenage BME school children in London have lower sexual health knowledge than white peers. Furthermore, within this sample, females had more sexual health knowledge than males, but the report stated that the difference in knowledge by ethnic groups is a major cause for concern. In relation to sexual experience, black Caribbean males were most likely to report having already had sex and Asian males the least likely. Almost half of the black Caribbean young men in the study reported having had underage sex; and 7% of these young men reported either getting their partner pregnant and/or acquiring an STI.

While the small numbers involved in the study mean that the statistical significance of the information needs to be viewed with some caution, the key issue here is that there is a need for sexual health support groups in BME communities, with a particular emphasis on black Caribbean young men. The findings of this study have been supported by other, larger scale reviews of the rates of STIs across ethnic groups and the reported relative use of genito-urinary services by men from different ethnic communities.[12,19-21]

This chapter will now focus on some of the specific sexual health issues pertaining to African, Caribbean and Asian men separately, as their experiences of sexual health differ greatly. In addition it is important to remember that planning and implementation of health promotion interventions need to take account of cultural and religious difference as a modifying factor in determining the appropriateness and effectiveness of the approach.[15,22] Each section will also include case examples of community-based interventions which have been successful in addressing the needs of men in these particular communities.

AFRICAN AND CARIBBEAN MEN

There have been a number of studies carried out investigating the prevalence of STIs in black men.[13,18,21] In general, what these studies have found is that, amongst black Caribbean and 'other' black groups, gonorrhoea can be up to 12–13 times higher, and chlamydia rates are nine times higher when compared with the majority 'white' population (http://www.kingsfund.org.uk). Much of these figures come from research conducted amongst the communities living in very ethnically diverse areas of London; however, similar patterns have been found in other parts of the UK and internationally.[23-25] In 2005 the Health Protection Agency (HPA) reported that gonorrhoea continues to affect black Caribbean communities disproportionately.[12] This evidence exists as further proof that the earlier sexual health campaigns which underpinned the 'Health of the Nation' strategies in the 1990s failed to make any significant impact on the sexual health of BME communities in the way they were publicised as meeting the targets for improving the sexual health of the nation as a whole.[26]

The British Survey of Sexual Attitudes and Lifestyles conducted in 2001 found that black African and black Caribbean men reported higher levels of sexual risk behaviour and higher incidence of STIs compared with white, Indian and Pakistani men.[27] There appeared to be varying factors as to why this could be, including the fact that the mean number of reported sexual partners in the last five years and a lifetime were highest amongst black Caribbean and African men. They also reported higher prevalence of concurrency in multiple partnerships and higher rates in partner acquisition. Other factors which appeared to impact on the levels of sexual ill health in this group included:

- The number of sex partners
- How partners were chosen
- Levels of untreated STIs generally in the community
- How quickly STIs were treated

Within all these areas, broader issues such as culture, age and marriage patterns were modifying factors across and within African and Caribbean community groups. Dr Fenton, who worked on the study, commented that the findings highlighted a need to work with communities to develop culturally appropriate approaches to STI prevention. His comments are supported by other studies in which it has been observed that gender roles and norms may influence STI risk behaviour of men and women within specific ethnic groups.[28–31]

A further consideration in the sexual health of African men and rates of untreated STIs in the community is the case of HIV and the African community. It is estimated that over 90% of heterosexually acquired HIV infections diagnosed in the UK during 2004 were probably acquired in high-prevalence countries of origin, mainly sub-Saharan Africa.[12] In addition, data from the UK and the Caribbean indicate that HIV rates are also increasing among black Caribbean communities.[28]

This chapter has already suggested that cultural norms and belonging to a minority ethnic group are not in themselves independent prerequisites for poor sexual health and increased risk of STIs. There are many compounding factors which, while not increasing the risk of infection per se, influence the health-seeking behaviours and decision making of African and Caribbean men in relation to their sexual health.[32]

One of the key factors is due to HIV-related stigma and discrimination which exist both in the country of origin and here in the UK. Research reports from the Caribbean, for example, suggest that, despite the increased knowledge about the causes and spread of STIs, many people still believe HIV to be a consequence and indication of homosexuality.[28] For many African men, they may be grappling with immigration issues and do not want to access services for fear of being 'caught' by immigration. Often the multiple problems on top of their immigration status, such as housing issues, isolation and mental health issues, can often mean that HIV is not considered as a pressing issue and may present as another problem to deal with. This short list represents only a quick snapshot of the catalogue of issues underpinning why many African and Caribbean men may not come forward to test their HIV or STI status.

Another key consideration in factors contributing to the higher rates of infection is accessing services. Again, a range of differing factors can influence this. For some African and Caribbean men who are new to the country, the whole system may be daunting. Appointment systems and drop-in, being unsure of your entitlements to free healthcare, in addition to any language barriers, can affect health-seeking behaviours. Broader issues relating to the ability of the service itself to address the needs of BME communities have long been highlighted in healthcare service reviews and patient satisfaction reports.[33,34] Deciding factors identified by patients and community service users as affecting their decision making include: Is it welcoming? Is there a diverse staff? Some people may or may not want to see someone from their own cultural background for fear of breaching confidentiality or embarrassment. Do the images on the wall reflect diversity? And is it male friendly? These may all have an impact on whether an individual decides to use a service, how quickly they perceive they will get treatment for an STI or HIV, and the overall appraisal of the quality of service by an ethnic group. The reported inability or unwillingness of some sexual health services to fulfil these requirements may be contributing factors to the higher rates of sexual ill health within African and Caribbean communities.[32]

It was mentioned earlier that recommendations have been made regarding culturally appropriate sexual health information for young people, particularly for boys from African and Caribbean communities. Currently the sex and relationships education (SRE) delivered in schools varies massively. Some schools have excellent comprehensive programmes that consider all the issues, whereas others provide the basics as part of a science lesson. This indicates large gaps for young people in their SRE; many then fill these gaps with information from friends, magazines, TV and other sources which are often myth based, incorrect and can leave them confused and feeling pressured. Below we present case studies of community-based sexual health programmes that have been successful in working with African and Caribbean men, particularly young men.

Project 1: Caribbean men – 'Awaredressers'

Background

The idea for this project came from an ongoing project in London of the same name. The project targeted businesses which are frequented by the West African community – originally being hairdressers, but the project has since extended to local food shops, restaurants and minicabs. The main aim was communication by the community members to raise awareness of HIV/AIDS, services and where to get free condoms. It also provides an opportunity to start the discussion of HIV and therefore tackles the stigma which still surrounds it.

Nottingham has a number of hairdressers and barbers that are a focal part of the African and African-Caribbean community. Long periods of time can be spent in the hairdressers and barbers and it can be quite a social environment, where discussions about a range of topics take place, including sex. Once the interested businesses were identified, a bid was made to the World AIDS Day Fund (WAD) 2002. The Awaredresser Project Leader in London was contacted early on to explain that we wanted to develop a sister project in Nottingham, which they were supportive of.

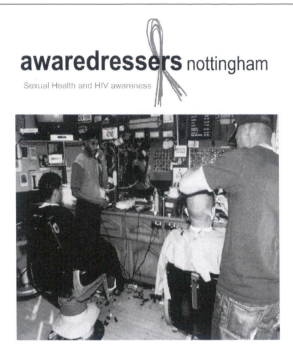

Figure 7.1: Awaredressers Nottingham.

Training was organised and hairdressers who had shown interest were invited. Only two hairdressers came along to the initial training event, with another member of staff. The training was well received and the participants all thought they had come away with some new information, as well as an understanding of the project. A second training course was planned but it had to be cancelled due to non-attendance. It was decided to go ahead with another three barbers and hairdressers even though they had not had training. The Awaredressers received condoms, sexual health leaflets, mugs, CD holders and World AIDS Day information, which they could leave out for their clients to take. The first evaluation was positive, and funding was sought from the Teenage Pregnancy Fund to continue.

The main functions of Awaredressers Nottingham are:

- To provide African-Caribbean barbers and hairdressers with condoms and sexual health information for their clients
- To raise awareness of sexual health and services in Nottingham
- To increase condom use among the African and Caribbean communities
- To gradually increase awareness about HIV/AIDS and start to address stigma and discrimination in the community

The project has grown in popularity and currently has 11 barbers and hairdressers involved. The current funding supports those in the NG7 area of Nottingham, and the other participants are supplied with condoms from previous funding. The project aims to add another two participants, hopefully African shops based in the Hyson Green area of Nottingham.

What has been observed over the past four years is that it takes time for the project to become established and known in the various shops. It was important for the project to engage with the black Caribbean communities as participants from

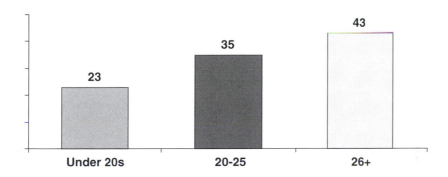

Figure 7.2: Clients accessing condoms by age group.

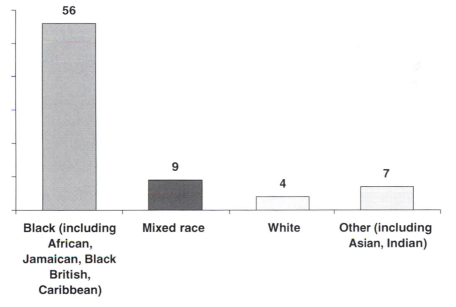

Figure 7.3: Clients accessing service by ethnic group.

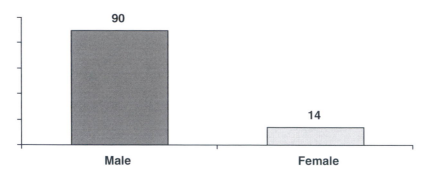

Figure 7.4: Clients accessing service by gender.

the beginning, as they are all well known to the community. It was also essential to have established a regular delivery time for condoms. At the time of writing, the newer businesses are still settling into the project and in the development stage, so clients may still be wary of taking the condoms. Indications are, however, that they will be as successful as the first cohort.

Figures 7.2–7.4 are compiled from figures from the monitoring sheets completed in three of the participating shops in 2004–2005. While the numbers are small (some people opted out of filling in the form), they indicate that the condoms were being predominantly accessed by the 'young' adult group of BME men, who were the main group targeted for this initiative.

The Awaredressers project is now in its fourth year. During that time money from both WAD and Teenage Pregnancy have funded it. More recently the project was successful in securing £5,000 from the New Deal for Communities, Community Support Fund.

This project has taken sexual health and access to condoms out of the traditional settings such as Contraception and Sexual Health clinics, genito-urinary medicine (GUM) and other sexual health projects, and placed it at a venue that is accessible, used regularly and accepted in the community. For black Caribbean men who may never have contact with the above services and may not be able to pay for condoms, this makes condoms easily accessible and free. Many free-condom projects only cater for a certain age group, while this is open to all men. The Awaredressers deal with varying clientele as far as age is concerned, and this can influence how quickly the condoms are taken.

Although monitoring has been difficult, we continue to put the forms in the shops and use whatever information we can from the completed sheets.

Box 7.1: Case studies

C The Barba – C's has the highest contact with the client group – young black men. The barber's is used often as a hang-out and the same faces are often around. The condom uptake here is very high, approximately 1,800 over three months. The barber felt that the shop is definitely a place to pick up condoms and a good way to promote sexual health in the black community. However, getting the young men to fill in the monitoring forms is more problematic; the barber felt that it did not make sense as the young men do not fill it out accurately. He continues to ask clients to fill out monitoring forms as it helps provide more funding for the project. He was asked if he would attend a sexual health session, but he thought it would be difficult to come out during business hours and obviously has personal business when not at work. The barber at C's is very vocal in promoting safer sex and has an area for posters.

Requests were made at this barber's for more Durex condoms and posters about the condoms; this has been followed through.

By visiting this barber regularly, it is easier to talk in the shop and some of the young men give their opinion on certain issues. This barber was also put into contact with Radio 1 Xtra through the project. They wanted to do a piece on barbers, including the involvement in the project.

C the Barba has since become part of the Awaredressers Management Committee and gives a valuable, on-the-ground perspective to the project and its future developments.

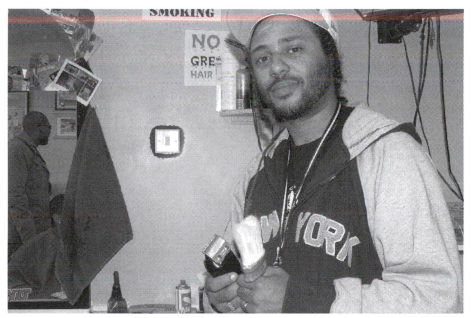

Figure 7.5: C the Barba.

Hi-Tek – Hi-Tek have been involved in Awaredressers Nottingham from the start. They were one of only two businesses that have taken part in Sexual Health/HIV training. Being a women's hairdresser's, the uptake of condoms is much slower but consistent. Condom drops to this hairdresser is approximately 4–6 months. There has been more success with the monitoring forms, although we cannot be sure of how correct the information is. The hairdresser was happy to continue in this project and felt that her business was known as a place to pick up condoms and sometimes leaflets. She also felt it was a good way to promote sexual health in the community.

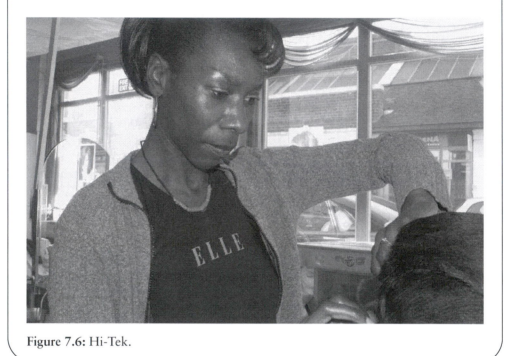

Figure 7.6: Hi-Tek.

Successes of the project

- Securing further funding to continue the project for at least the next year and setting up a Management Committee
- Retaining three of the original Awaredressers, who are now established and known as part of the project
- Increases in condom uptake in those businesses who have been involved for two years or more
- Recognition of the project within the community at large
- That the project is doing what it was set up to do

Challenges

- To encourage monitoring at each participating business
- To involve the Awaredressers in some sort of training or awareness-raising around sexual health and the communities so they can feel more confident around the issues
- To continue to secure funding to sustain and develop this project

The project has challenged myths and stereotypes that surround black men and their sexual health. It has demonstrated that they will use condoms but often the problem is around accessibility of condoms. You either have to be under 18 years old or feel confident using a sexual health service to access free condoms, otherwise you pay for them, and condoms are often not a priority when you have limited funds. It also gives us a platform to promote campaigns such as Sexual Health Week and World AIDS Day, and in the past additional resources have been produced such as mugs and calendars featuring health education messages and the participant businesses from Awaredressers. The calendars were handed out to clients and have kept the HIV/safer sex message on walls throughout the year, as well as featuring all those involved. This has been very successful and will hopefully be continued each year.

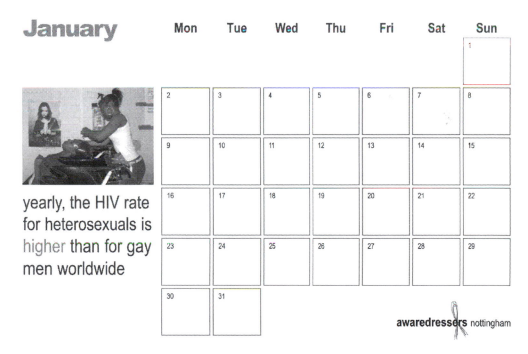

Figure 7.7: Example of Awaredressers calendar.

Project 2: African men

Box 7.2: Case Study – Beyond Condom Campaign

The Beyond Condom Campaign is a national campaign being led by the National African HIV Prevention Programme (NAHIP), developed by the Black Health Agency. It uses the slogan 'Let's talk HIV – Let's Talk Safer Sex' to encourage the African community to increase condom use, but also to begin to talk about issues around sex and HIV. Because the African community is extremely diverse, this has to be done in a way that is compatible with various cultural and religious practices. The project has a three-year span.

The campaign has developed a range of posters and leaflets targeting people living with HIV, sexually active adults and men who have sex with men.

The campaign has set out guidelines for how the promotion may take place. In Nottingham the focus is on the outreach part of the campaign, which will involve volunteers from the African community disseminating the leaflets by having contact with individuals at events such as Carnival or market days. The posters will be put up in local businesses, community centres and other places the community utilises.

In Nottingham the Beyond Condom Campaign is led by a voluntary organisation – African Initiative Support – with support from a member of the Positive Care Team and Health Promotion Unit. The volunteers are mostly of African origin, predominantly men, have refugee or asylum-seeking status and speak more than one language. To prepare the volunteers we have put on a number of sessions that have taken them through the basics around HIV, condom use, the campaign and what their role is, but importantly building their confidence and preparing them for going out and talking to members of their community about an issue that is often taboo and not discussed.

The sessions have been very successful, and we are preparing the volunteers to go out and do their first outreach session at the annual Carnival event in 2006.

Success (so far ...)

- Positive response from the volunteers, who have attended the weekly two-hour sessions and participated well
- Growing confidence in the volunteers, along with a passion for HIV prevention and wanting to help the community
- A passionate and committed project leader
- Potential for another training course and more volunteers

Challenges (so far ...)

- Lack of female volunteers that could address gender difficulties, i.e. men speaking to women about sex

- Numbers have varied over the weeks we have put on the sessions, with about five core volunteers attending each one. This could be due to other unforeseen situations that prevented them attending all the sessions
- We foresee challenges when the volunteers start to go out into the community. These hopefully will be dealt with through continuing support sessions and addressing issues as they come up

ASIAN MEN

As mentioned previously the sexual health issues and needs of BME men vary greatly. Among Asian communities talking about sex is generally seen as taboo, so these discussions are not often had at home. Combined with possible poor sex and relationships education (SRE) in school or being removed from the subject by their parents in schools, some Asian people have had no formal information about sexual health and perhaps do not get that information from friends in the same way other young people might. Through her research and work with Asian young people, Kanwaljit Bhogal (health promotion specialist – Asian young people and sexual health) found that young people wanted more information and somewhere safe to go when seeking advice and support. Through group work with Pakistani young men, Kanwaljit managed to tap into some of their feelings around sex and relationships. A summary of the topics discussed and issues highlighted are shown in Figure 7.8.

There were some interesting insights from this piece of work, such as themes around not talking about sex, high emphasis placed on marriage and the perceptions of young Asian women.

Stereotypes and assumptions about BME communities regarding sex and relationships often dictate how they may be perceived within services.[32] For people from Asian communities, for example, assumptions that arranged marriages can be seen more as forced marriages, and that young Asian people do not have sex before marriage and therefore STIs and pregnancy are not an issue for them, are some of the general beliefs that often dictate the nature or availability of sexual health information and services provided.

Research has shown that there is a higher level of sexual abstinence among Asians, particularly women, and an underreporting of condom use by Asian men,[21] which poses the question of whether existing services are carrying out appropriate sexual health promotion and information that support the sexual lifestyles of Asian people.

There is currently limited research into Asian men and sexual health. The Naz Project London has carried out some research specifically into the needs of South Asian men who have sex with men. Other statistics and pieces of research around sexual health show that Asian populations have a lower incidence of STIs and HIV, although it is recognised that this needs to be monitored because of the increases in HIV prevalence across Asia.[12]

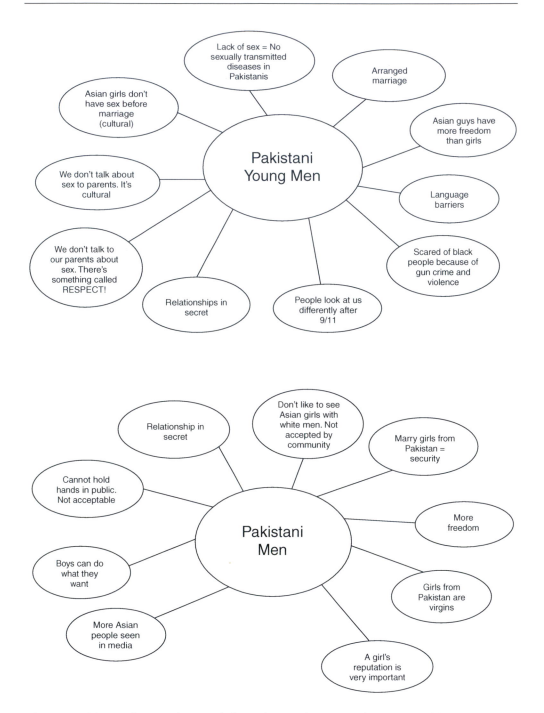

Figure 7.8: Topics discussed in workshops during the men-only time (MOT) event.

Parminda Sekon from the Naz Project explained that many people of South Asian origin found it impossible to admit their HIV status and were reluctant to admit how they had contracted the disease. 'I think there is a huge problem for people about how they will be treated if they disclose their status and the stigma and prejudice they will face', she said, adding that this was driving HIV underground in certain Asian communities. 'People have popular perceptions about how this is transmitted and they are things like pre-marital and extra-marital sex, things that are considered taboo in these communities'.

She said that this often resulted in people being reluctant to admit they had contracted the disease through sexual transmissions. In addition, the backlash against homosexuality within many communities made it especially difficult for married South Asian gay men, who were often left with little alternative but to continue living double lives.[36]

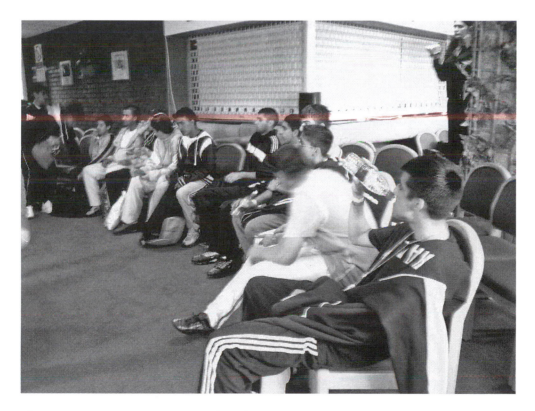

Figure 7.9: Young Asian men attending the MOT event.

Box 7.3: Case Study – men-only time (MOT) event

The aim of this event was to raise awareness of sexual health among South Asian young men in a holistic way. The event brought Pakistani, Indian and Bangladeshi young men together, although the majority who attended were from a Pakistani background. The age span was from 12 to 19 years and the young men came from across Nottingham.

The sexual health work was carried out through workshops and theatre production, which was an interactive piece with a scenario that focussed on a young Asian girl who is pregnant, her partner and his mother. Discussions focussed on the positive reaction of the boyfriend's mother to the pregnancy. The young men responded and interacted well with the drama piece.

In the workshop three questions were presented to the young men:

Question 1:
Your best friend Romy, who is 16, confides in you that he is thinking about having sex with his girlfriend.
What advice would you give him?

Question 2:
A young Asian boy wants to get some free condoms. He does not want to go to the Victoria Health Centre.
Where could he go?
Where would be the ideal place to get free condoms?
Who would be the ideal person to give them to him?

Question 3:
Men are always the ones who start any kind of sexual advances in a relationship.

This gave the young men an opportunity to explore some of the issues related to sexual health.

Kanwaljit concluded that:
If the barrier is high for young men in general when accessing services, how high is this barrier for young South Asian men? We need to build confidence and self-esteem so young men can be empowered to take responsibility for their sexual health, as well as imparting information so they can make informed decisions in relation to sexual health and their beliefs. I believe it is so important to ensure South Asian young men are involved in designing services, and have the opportunity to 'mystery shop' these services.

Overall the evaluation by the young men was very positive; many felt that it should be done more often. They enjoyed the workshops and the opportunity to discuss the issues and gain new information.

Successes of the project

- Beginnning to present sex and relationship issues and open them up for discussion in a way that has been acceptable to young people, particularly young men
- Based on the positive reception of the drama piece, there is a further Theatre in Education project being developed to continue the theme of teenage pregnancy and sexual health, presented in a way that is culturally appropriate and acceptable to young Asian people
- Working in partnership with the youth service and other organisations to bring as many young men together and put on the event

Challenges of project

- Ending of the Asian Young People and Sexual Health post affected capacity and continuation of this work
- Some reluctance by youth workers to be involved in sexual health work, which then has an influence on how this work is taken forward
- Issues on the day around female Asian workers delivering sexual health workshops; however, due to the point above, it is difficult to find a trained Asian man to deliver sexual health education

THE WAY FORWARD

Throughout this chapter varying issues for BME men and their sexual health have been explored. The key requirements underpinning all the issues highlighted is the need for BME men to have their sexual health needs met while being treated with cultural and religious considerations in mind.

There seems to be a case for a much better comprehensive SRE programme to be run in schools, one that takes into consideration other religions and cultures as an influencing factor on sexual health behaviour, that presents the emotional issues arising from minority ethnic experience alongside STIs/HIV, and that is able to talk about sex within a relationship. Discussions of sexual health in single-sex groups need to be considered to enable young men and women to express themselves and gain the information they need without being embarrassed.

There are significant differences in the sexual health of BME groups. This will influence the way health-promotion initiatives are developed. In the experiences of those highlighted in the case studies, taking the sexual health and condoms to the men has been working. It is difficult to quantitatively prove that this is reducing teenage pregnancy and STIs, but what it does show is that condoms are being accessed, hopefully used and that information is travelling through word of mouth.

With Asian communities it seems important to continue to present sexual health in a holistic way, perhaps as part of a Men's Day, residential or through theatre, where there is not an obvious emphasis on sexual health but it is a major part of the event. The young men attending these events have evaluated positively and expressed an interest in these events being ongoing, also appreciating the opportunity to talk about sexual health issues.

As the African community continues to grow and become more established, there will be opportunities to work more and more through community groups that are set up and community events that celebrate African culture. The emphasis will be around HIV, condom use and testing as these are the major sexual health issues that affect that community. It is also important to involve churches as they can be a central source of support for individuals who may be facing a number of problems, HIV being just one.

To build on and develop work with BME men, it is essential that good quality research continues to be carried out not only in London but in other parts of the country, to allow evidence-based health promotion and sexual health practice to be continually developed.

Although there is government recognition of the problems that face BME communities through the National Sexual Health and HIV Strategy, The Teenage Pregnancy Strategy and more recently Choosing Health, it is vital that locally the voluntary, statutory and community organisations work in partnership to reduce teenage pregnancy, reduce STIs and HIV, provide quality SRE, and offer support to parents and carers in talking to their children about sex.

Improving the sexual health of men from BME communities is a complex task. It involves engaging with many difficult subjects and integrating a clearer understanding of the cultural and ethnic diversity within and between communities. This chapter can only hope to begin to give an insight into the range of issues involved. If it has managed to highlight the concerns and encourage further research, discussion and action in this arena, it will have achieved its goal.

REFERENCES

1 Sewell T. A phallic response to schooling – black masculinity and race in an inner city comprehensive. In: Griffiths M and Troyna B, editors. *Antiracism, culture and social justice in education.* Stoke-on-Trent: Trentham Books; 1995. Chapter 2.
2 Whitehead S. Masculinities, race and nationhood – critical connections. *Gend Hist* 2000; **12**(2): 472–476.
3 Gibbs JT. *Young, black and male in America: an endangered species.* Dover, MA: Auburn House; 1988.
4 Office for National Statistics. *The health of adult Britain 1891–1994.* London: The Stationery Office; 1997.
5 Khunti K and Farooqi A. Diabetes. In: Kai J, editor. *Ethnicity, health and primary care.* Oxford: Oxford University Press; 2003. pp. 113–121.

6 Patel S. Mental health. In: Kai J, editor. *Ethnicity, health and primary care*. Oxford: Oxford University Press; 2003. pp. 131–139.

7 Hussein RG. The health care and health status of ethno-cultural minorities in the United Kingdom: an agenda for action. *J Adv Nurs* 1995; **21**(2): 199–201.

8 Nazroo JY. *Ethnicity, class and health*. London: Policy Studies Institute; 2001.

9 Macbeth H and Shetty P, editors. *Health and ethnicity*. London: Taylor and Francis; 2001.

10 Karlsen S and Nazroo JY. Agency and structure: The impact of ethnic identity and racism on the health of ethnic minority people. *Sociol Health Illn* 2002; **24**(1): 1–20.

11 Adams J. Sex and politics. In: McAndews S, editor. *Sexual health – foundations for practice*. London: Baillière Tindall/RCN; 2000. pp. 33–45.

12 Health Protection Agency. *HIV and other sexually transmitted infections in the UK*. London: HPA; 2005.

13 Fenton K and Wellings K. Sexual health and ethnicity. In: Macbeth H and Shetty P, editors. *Health and ethnicity*. London: Taylor and Francis; 2001. pp. 223–232.

14 Geringer WM, Marks S, Allen WJ and Armstrong KA. Knowledge, attitudes and behaviour related to condom use and STDs in a high risk population. *J Sex Res* 1993; **30**(1): 75–83.

15 Balsa A and McGuire T. Prejudice, clinical uncertainty and stereotyping as sources of health disparities. *J Health Econ* 2003; **22**: 89–116.

16 Culley L. A critique of multiculturalism in health care: the challenge for nurse education. *J Adv Nurs* 1996; **23**(3): 564–570.

17 Gerrish K, Husband C and Mackenzie J. *Nursing for a multi-ethnic society*. Buckingham: Open University Press; 1996.

18 Low N, Daker-White G, Barlow D and Pozniak AL. Gonorrhoea in inner London: results of a cross-sectional survey. *BMJ* 1997; **314**: 1719–1723.

19 Fenton K, Johnson AM and Nicoll A. Race, ethnicity and sexual health. *BMJ* 1997; **314**(June): 1703–1706.

20 Wellings K, Field J, Johnson A and Wadsworth J. *Sexual behaviour in Britain*. London: Penguin; 1994.

21 Lacey CJN, Merrick DW, Bensley DC and Fairley I. Analysis of the sociodemographics of gonorrhoea in Leeds, 1989–93. *BMJ* 1997; **314**: 1715–1718.

22 Kai J, editor. *Ethnicity, health and primary care*. Oxford: Oxford University Press; 2003.

23 Cock KM de and Low N. HIV and AIDS, other sexually transmitted diseases and tuberculosis in ethnic minorities in the United Kingdom: is surveillance serving its purpose? *BMJ* 1997; **314**: 1747–1751.

24 Crepaz N and Marks G. Towards an understanding of sexual risk behaviour in people living with HIV: a review of social, psychological and medical findings. *AIDS* 2002; **16**(2): 135–149.

25 Blum R, Beuring T, Shew M, Bearinger L, Sieving R and Rensick M. The effects of race/ethnicity, income and family structure on adolescent risk behaviors. *Am J Public Health* 2000; **90**(12): 1879–1884.

26 Adler MW. Sexual health – A health of the nation failure. *BMJ* 1997; **314**: 1743–1747.

27 Johnson A, Mercer CH, Erens B, Copas AJ, McManus S, Wellings K, *et al.* Sexual behaviour in Britain: partnerships, practices and HIV risk behaviours. *Lancet* 2001; **358**: 1835–1842.

28 Kempadoo K. Freelancers, temporary wives and beach-boys: researching sex work in the Caribbean. *Feminist Rev* 2001; **67**(Spring): 39–62.

29 Rothenberg R. How a net works: implications of network structure for the persistence and control of sexually transmitted diseases and HIV. *Sex Transm Dis* 2001; **28**(2): 63–68.

30 Santelli J, Lowry R, Brener N and Robin L. The association of sexual behaviors with socioeconomic status, family structure and race/ethnicity among US adolescents. *Am J Public Health* 2000; **90**(10): 1582–1588.

31 Sionean C, DiClimente R, Wingood G, Crosby R, Cobb B, Harrington K, *et al.* Socioeconomic status and self-reported gonorrhoea among African American female adolescents. *Sex Transm Dis* 2001; **28**(4): 236–239.

32 Serrant-Green L. *Black Caribbean men, sexual health decisions and silences*. PhD Thesis. Nottingham: University of Nottingham; 2004.

33 Department of Health. *The national strategy for sexual health and HIV*. London: DoH; 2001.

34 Department of Health. *Effective commissioning of sexual health and HIV services*. London: DoH; 2003.

35 Testa A, Coleman L and Naz Project London. *Sexual health knowledge, attitudes and behaviours among Black and minority ethnic youth in London*. London: The Trust for the Study of Adolescence; 2006.

36 BBC News 2003. China launches sex website. Retrieved 26/02/04 from http://news.bbc.co.uk/go/pr/fr/-/hi/world/asia-pacific/3059267.stm

CHAPTER 8

Providing sexual health services for men

Kevin Miles

> **Key points**
>
> A range of innovative, culturally appropriate and co-ordinated approaches are required to provide accurate service provision for men.
>
> Sexual health services should empower and involve male service users in decision making.
>
> There is a need for better information about the range of sexual health services available to men, with male-targeted media playing a bigger role.

INTRODUCTION

The National Teenage Pregnancy Strategy[1] and *National Strategy for Sexual Health and HIV*[2] have placed the provision of services for sexual health and HIV high on the political agenda for the first time ever. These strategies aim to:

- Reduce the transmission of HIV and sexually transmitted infections (STIs)
- Reduce the prevalence of undiagnosed HIV and STIs
- Reduce unintended pregnancy rates
- Improve health and social care for people living with HIV
- Reduce the stigma associated with HIV and STIs

A number of other documents have followed in order to provide strategic direction for prevention, service provision, commissioning and a range of other necessary requirements to support change.[3–5] Also supporting these strategies, the *National*

115

Service Framework for Children, Young People and Maternity Services[6] and *Every Child Matters: Change for Children*[7] set standards for health promotion and prevention in young people to reduce the risk of both teenage pregnancy and acquiring an STI.

The culmination of sexual health strategic direction, and a demonstration of the high level of political commitment for improving sexual health, is the Government's public health white paper, *Choosing Health: Making Healthy Choices Easier.*[8] Of the five priority areas for improving public health, *Choosing Health* outlined proposals for a national campaign targeted particularly at younger men and women to ensure that they understand the real risk of unprotected sex and to persuade them of the benefits of using condoms to avoid the risk of STIs or unplanned pregnancies. This document also set service targets, including:

- By March 2007, a national screening programme for chlamydia will cover all areas of England
- By 2008, patients referred to a genito-urinary medicine (GUM) clinic will be able to have an appointment within 48 hours

As such, there is now increased pressure for organisations to provide faster access to sexual health services, for more individuals, in more different settings. Professionals involved in delivering sexual health services come from a range of backgrounds, including health, education and social sectors, set within a variety of public (NHS), voluntary, community and independent settings. Although this chapter will attempt to address the role of sexual health services for men across these various backgrounds and settings, it will primarily focus on sexual health services within the public health sector.

POLICY RHETORIC AND SEXUAL HEALTH SERVICES FOR MEN

Recent sexual health policy developments in Britain have focussed on adverse outcomes of sexual behaviour, such as STIs, including HIV, and unintended pregnancy. Furthermore, STI screening has been focussed on women, as infections such as chlamydia are a major cause of pelvic inflammatory disease, ectopic pregnancy and infertility. For this reason, research, health promotion and disease prevention initiatives have focussed mainly on women. This is in spite of a substantial body of evidence reporting that men have an equal, if not greater, risk of acquiring sexual infections than women. Specific services for men who have sex with men (MSM) have been developed in line with the high prevalence of STIs and HIV in this population, but in general there has been a distinct failure in national policy to identify any means by which the sexual health needs of the heterosexual male population can be equally targeted. It has been argued that the failure to address the sexual health needs of heterosexual men is a human rights issue.

Targeting heterosexual men comes with its own problems; a key reason why men have been neglected in national STI screening policy and planning. There are significant differences in health-seeking behaviours and existing levels of service access for heterosexual men and women. Whilst women regularly access general practice and other primary care services in order to receive ongoing contraception and have routine cervical cytology smears performed, men have less of an immediate need to attend services for preventive health reasons. Women also tend to be more concerned when they experience genital symptoms, with a vested interest in future reproductive health; whereas men often portray avoidance attitudes and behaviours.[9] Where men's symptoms are vague, they often do not recognise the importance of their symptoms and assume things will get better. When they do acknowledge their symptoms, more than a third will continue to have sex.[10] Many men will have relatively poor knowledge of where to go, and a sudden decision to access services is often followed by frustration in obtaining an appointment.[11]

As a result, it is easier and more pragmatic to target women through existing service networks than it is for men. The main screening locations for the National Chlamydia Screening Programme in England have included: contraception clinics, young people's services, gynaecology departments, antenatal services, colposcopy services, termination of pregnancy services, and general practice – the majority of these being identified as services for women. Consequently, the first two years of the programme found that men accounted for only 11% of the 80,000 screens performed, and yet the positivity rate was higher in men than women (11.7% compared with 10.9%).[12]

WHAT CONSTITUTES A SEXUAL HEALTH SERVICE?

In order to define sexual health services for men, it is important to reflect on the definition of sexual health. Sexual health is not just about STIs, HIV and unintended pregnancy. The concept of sexual health is broad in its definition, including elements of sexual relationships, sexual fulfillment, sexual identity, illness, disease and unintended pregnancy,[2,13,14] yet national policy and local services are mostly restricted to the identification and management of illness and disease. As a result, not all sexual health services will be able to fulfil the needs of the community with regard to achieving what has been defined as 'good sexual health'. Different services will provide different elements of sexual health care, and this is largely dependent on the type of organisation providing services (e.g. public versus independent) and the associated objectives, physical infrastructure, human resource capacity and capability, and funding arrangements. In addition, traditional vertical approaches to service provision have resulted in 'silo working', whereby a variety of services each provide one element of sexual healthcare, with little co-ordination between them. For instance, to date, most contraception and GUM service providers have worked independently from each other, even though they are mostly providing an element of sexual healthcare for the same sexually active population. As a result opportunities for STI screening in contraception services have been missed, as have opportunities to address contraception in GUM attenders.

Furthermore, sexual difficulties in men are widely prevalent in the general population. The most recent British estimates come from Natsal 2000, a stratified probability sample survey conducted between May 1999 and February 2001 of 11,161 men and women aged 16–44 years, resident in Britain.[15] A total of 34.8% of men who had at least one heterosexual partner in the previous year reported at least one sexual problem lasting at least one month during this period.[16] The most common problems among men were lack of interest in sex, premature orgasm and anxiety about performance. However, in terms of sexual health policy, relatively little attention has been paid to sexual fulfilment or function, despite their strong association with quality of life.

Where non-STI-related sexual health services are provided, they may be restricted in what they can offer. For example, GUM services may be able to provide assessment for sexual dysfunction, but may have to refer patients to general practitioners (GPs) or independent or voluntary providers for psychosexual and/or pharmacotherapy intervention. This is not an optimal scenario given that a man may have taken some time to build the courage to seek care for his sexual dysfunction, only to find that he needs further referral, or has to disclose his condition to the family doctor. In essence, there are relatively few one-stop sexual health services for men that address all of the elements incorporated in the definition of sexual health and well-being.

The clearest evidence demonstrating the lack of attention to men's sexual health can be seen within the three levels of sexual health services that were defined by the *National Strategy for Sexual Health and HIV*.[2]

Level one sexual health service providers have been defined as GPs with an interest in sexual health. At this level women are able to access STI testing and yet men can only be assessed and referred. Many patients initially attend GP services for STIs before being managed by GUM services, and primary care is therefore already an important setting, with potential for STI control. This undoubtedly represents a missed opportunity for men to be screened and treated for STIs.

However, it is likely that over time this inequality will be overcome, as the evidence stacks against leaving men out of the equation. Delivering at all of these levels as it stands is a challenge in itself, but providers need to be open to directing resources where they are best placed to meet the needs of the local population. This is likely to take some time and be complicated by the ever-changing political landscape. Health sector reform, including payment by results, practice-based commissioning and the general trend for the NHS to become less of a direct service provider and more of a service commissioner will all affect sexual services provision at each of the aforementioned levels of care.

Box 8.1: Sexual health services

Level One:
- sexual history and risk assessment
- STI testing for women
- HIV testing and counselling
- pregnancy testing and referral
- contraceptive information and services
- assessment and referral of men with STI symptoms
- cervical cytology screening and referral
- hepatitis B immunisation

Level Two:
- intrauterine device (IUD) insertion
- testing and treating STIs
- vasectomy
- contraceptive implant insertion
- partner notification
- invasive STI
- testing for men (until non-invasive tests are available)

Level Three: Level three clinician teams will take responsibility for sexual health services needs-assessment, for supporting provider quality, for clinical governance requirements at all levels and for providing specialist services. Services could include:
- outreach for STI prevention
- outreach contraception services
- specialised infections management, including co-ordination of partner notification
- highly specialised contraception
- specialised HIV treatment and care

Finally, whilst these levels of care are still largely centred on STIs, HIV and unintended pregnancy, there are common principles that apply across any service. The Medical Foundation for AIDS and Sexual Health (MedFASH) recommended that people should receive a service which:

- Is service-user centred
- Enables self-referral to services
- Encourages partnership in decision-making
- Enables them to make informed and autonomous choices
- Supports them in taking responsibility for their sexual health care

This means that people need to have access to clear information about where local services are, what they can offer and how they can be accessed. This may involve advertising in non-traditional settings such as the workplace or sport and recreation facilities. The public will also have an increasing role in determining what services should be on offer in the future. Whether these acts of devolution and increased user involvement will provide dividends for the broader sexual healthcare of men is to be seen.

WHAT DO MAINSTREAM STATUTORY SEXUAL HEALTH SERVICES OFFER?

Genito-urinary medicine clinics

GUM clinics have been the mainstay of sexual health services for men since their inception in the post-Royal Commission era following World War One.[17] Men now account for approximately 48% of all GUM clinic workload, which increased from 263,108 male patients in 1999 to 680,729 in 2003.[18]

NHS GUM services are unique in that they have a legal duty to secure patient information.[19] This means that patients can attend a GUM service with confidence that partners, insurance companies and other healthcare providers cannot access their information.

There are over 200 GUM clinics in the UK providing free and confidential services that can be accessed by any individual without the need for referral. GUM services are provided by a multidisciplinary team of doctors, nurses, health advisers, administration and support staff. Some GUM teams include clinical psychologists and other allied health and social care professionals. Clinics will vary as to whether they provide an appointment-based service, walk-in or mix of both.

The main remit of a GUM clinic is to identify and manage STIs, including HIV. The usual care pathway through a GUM clinic includes an asessment of the individual's symptoms and sexual behaviour, followed by a physical assessment and collection of specimens from relevant genital sites. GUM clinics have unique rapid diagnostic ability, as some of the genital samples can be viewed under an on-site microscope to provide an immediate indication of infection. Treatment is provided free of charge and supplied at the point of care.

GUM clinics also provide a range of specialist services that can include:

- Same-day, or point-of-care (within the hour) HIV testing
- Post-exposure prophylaxis following sexual exposure to HIV (PEPSE)
- Sexual assault services
- Sexual dysfunction clinics
- Chronic genital problem clinics (e.g. recurrent herpes, persistent warts, genital dermatoses)
- Hepatitis clinics

- Psychosexual counselling
- Designated clinics for target groups
- Outreach clinics for target groups

In terms of clinical management, GUM clinics have followed a traditional approach to care for some time, with GUM physicians leading on all consultations, supported by nursing and allied staff. However, with technology advances, changing service-user needs and demands, shifting professional roles and increased pressure to deliver better value for money, novel approaches to improving the patient experience are being developed.

A range of practitioners are now leading on patient consultations, enabling more services to be offered in a range of GUM and non-GUM clinical settings. Nurse-led clinics have become increasingly popular[20] and research has demonstrated these to be safe and effective, with high levels of patient satisfaction.[21–24]

Services are also reconfiguring care pathways that enable faster access and faster throughput, such as the 'test not talk' (TNT) service for men that spends minimal time gathering information from the patient and performs a minimal set of tests.[25] The use of technology is being exploited to improve the acceptability and uptake of STI testing, in particular the use of urine testing for chlamydia in young men. New ways to provide results are also exploiting information, technology and communication systems, therefore reducing the need to re-attend services. The use of mobile phone text-messaging services is becoming increasingly popular and can increase patient satisfaction, reduce staff workload and reduce the time to treatment.[26–28]

Box 8.2: General sexual health sources of information for men

- The Family Planning Association (fpa) provides confidential information and advice on contraception and sexual and reproductive health, and details of sexual health services anywhere in the UK: http://www.fpa.org.uk
- The British Association for Sexual Health & HIV provides professionals with information, including clinical guidelines for the management of STIs and other sexual health problems: http://www.bashh.org
- The British Association for Sexual and Relationship Therapy provides a list of UK therapists: http://www.basrt.org.uk
- Relate provides therapy for sex problems: http://www.relate.org.uk
- The Sexual Dysfunction Association provides public and professionals with information about sexual problems: http://www.sda.uk.net

---

Contraception services

Traditionally, responsibility for both using contraception and dealing with any consequent problems has been seen as 'women's business'. Sex and relationship education in schools and from parents and carers has focussed on protecting women from the consequences of sexual activity; contraceptive services have been provided almost exclusively by and for women; and women and men themselves have viewed men as peripheral to preventing unwanted pregnancy.

Data on how men use contraception services is limited. This is partly the case for women also, in that detailed information about routine use of services is currently only available from NHS family planning clinics and Brook Advisory Centres. Within these providers about 1.2 million female and 91,000 male atendances were recorded in 2001–2002.[29] Although the number of male attendances constitute a very small percentage of the total attenders, the number has more than doubled since 1991–1992. This implies a changing trend in male reproductive health-seeking behaviours, although[30] it suggests that most of this increase is due to more men obtaining condoms. A significant proportion of men attend contraception services for vasectomy, although the estimated 45,000–50,000 vasectomies that are performed each year have remained constant since the early 1980s.[29] Further contraceptive services are also provided by GPs, hospitals, voluntary organisations and by the private sector, but detailed information about male use is limited.

Nonetheless, there is a new cultural shift in developing an understanding about why men act as they do, how they utilise services and what their needs are. To support the Teenage Pregnancy Strategy,[1] *Guidance for developing contraception and sexual health advice services to reach boys and young men*[31] set out to encourage contraception services to make special efforts to increase the uptake by boys and young men. Suggested interventions included involving boys and young men in needs analysis, providing targeted services in male-friendly settings such as sports institutions and barber shops, and monitoring and evaluating uptake of services by men.

Despite the increasing emphasis on male involvement in family planning and a greater acceptance for men to be trusted to shoulder this responsibility, choices for contraception continue to be directed at women. Apart from condom use and vasectomy, there have been no advances in male-controlled contraception methods in the last century. Hormonal contraceptives for men are still in the clinical research stages, with promises of new methods forever 'just around the corner'.[32] Finding a new male-focussed method has the potential to revolutionise reproductive health choices, but until then services can only continue to engage men in proactively supporting their female partners with the current female contraceptive choices.

Secondary care services

Urology services, and to a degree fertility services, are also involved in the care of men with sexual health problems and conditions. Urologists manage a range of sexual health issues, including investigating and managing non-STI genital conditions such as prostadynia, recurrent urethritis and erectile dysfunction. They may also be involved in performing gender reassignment. They usually require referral and are mostly located within the acute sector hospitals. Urology services are also available in the independent sector.

TARGETED SEXUAL HEALTH SERVICES FOR MEN

Adolescent men

STIs are a major public health problem in people aged 16–24 years. In 2003, young men aged 16–24 accounted for 55% of all chlamydia diagnoses in men, 41% of gonorrhoea and 44% of genital warts diagnosed in GUM clinics in England, Wales and Northern Ireland.[33] However, a common problem is that young men lack accurate information about STI transmission and acquisition, prevention methods, signs and symptoms, and how and when to access services. Although STI and HIV awareness has improved over time, peer beliefs, attitudes and behaviours can override sensible judgement and fuel elements of stigma, shame and embarrassment.

Young men also lack information and good role models on how to conduct themselves as sexual beings. The media is overloaded with highly sexualised images that tend to set the norm for what growing up is all about. The pressure for adolescent men to be sexual and prove their manhood before they are actually aware and ready to accept the associated consequences and responsibilities can lead to a multitude of problems. Whilst the media, parents, carers and society in general have a responsibility to address this, services also play a crucial role. Service providers have a responsibility to positively and proactively target young men and boys, and address issues not only about STIs and contraception, but also puberty, masturbation, self-esteem, relationships, testicular cancer, same-sex feelings, sex and the law, sexual assault and rape, and parenting and fatherhood. Interventions should not be restricted to improving knowledge and awareness: skills development set within the context of clarifying beliefs and perceptions, and addressing attitudes, motivations and intentions, is integral to developing or modifying personal behaviour.

In setting up sexual health services for boys and young men, providers should consider how they could increase the direct involvement of their future 'service users'. The use of focus groups is one way that can help develop a greater understanding of the needs of male clients.[34] Taking on such initiatives needs creativity in order to identify the target population and attract them in to provide their views and opinions. In terms of evaluating services, there is a need for more innovative approaches beyond satisfaction questionnaires, such as the Undercover Youth Participation initiative that has adopted a 'mystery shopper'-style approach to evaluation.[35] Any new development should have core elements of monitoring and evaluation incorporated to ensure that outcomes are achieved alongside value for money.

In terms of providing contraception and sexual health services for adolescent men, notably those under the age of 16, there are specific issues that services need to address. These primarily relate to the ability for a young person to provide consent to receive treatment or advice about sexual health, without the consent of a parent or legal guardian. To deal with this the Department of Health has provided guidance that doctors and other health professionals should follow when dealing with under 16s.[36] The key points include:

- Health professionals have a duty of care and a duty of confidentiality to all patients, including under-16s
- All services providing contraceptive advice and treatment to young people should:
  - Produce an explicit confidentiality policy, making clear that under-16s have the same right to confidentiality as adults
  - Prominently advertise services as confidential for young people under 16, within the service and in community settings where young people meet

The duty of confidentiality is not, however, absolute. Where a health professional believes that there is a risk to the health, safety or welfare of a young person or others which is so serious as to outweigh the young person's right to privacy, they should follow locally agreed child-protection protocols.

In order to be able to deem under-16s competent to make their own decisions, it is considered good practice for health professionals to follow the criteria outlined by Lord Fraser in 1985. These were originally developed for the provision of contraception, but have generally been adopted to assess all under-16s when providing sexual health services, including the provision of condoms, information and STI screening and treatment. These are commonly known as the Fraser Guidelines:

- The young person understands the health professional's advice
- The health professional cannot persuade the young person to inform his or her parents or allow the doctor to inform the parents that he or she is seeking contraceptive advice
- The young person is very likely to begin or continue having intercourse with or without contraceptive treatment
- Unless he or she receives contraceptive advice or treatment, the young person's physical or mental health or both are likely to suffer
- The young person's best interests require the health professional to give contraceptive advice, treatment or both without parental consent

Young men's sexual health information and awareness interventions have mostly been led by community-based organisations (CBOs), some in partnership with local schools and some with mainstream sexual health services. Some CBOs and GUM clinics have also jointly provided sexual health services (STI screening, diagnosis and treatment) in community-based 'outreach' or 'satellite' settings. These have been met with varying success.

Despite the right motivations, young persons' services do not always need to be set within community spaces. Success in mainstream services has been proven, but difficulties lay in these interventions also, and therefore they do not provide the only solution. Difficulties in running mainstream services for young men-only include meeting the sometimes competing needs of young women and young men. Young men are poorer attenders than young women, can be disruptive (particularly in large groups) and can display inappropriate behaviour towards female clients and female members of staff. Hancock[83] suggests possible solutions for this include having the right workers, providing the right training, overcoming time and space problems, and offering information and easier access to condoms. Hancock also suggests that a dual approach is probably needed, where specialist male-only services are run alongside mainstream services, either within the same space or in outreach settings.

Where services are provided in outreach settings, clinical practices may need to change to reflect the environment and available resources. On-site microscopy, which can support an immediate clinical diagnosis, may not be available. In such instances professionals should consider syndromic management approaches. This can lead to an overuse of antibiotics, but, given the high prevalence of infections such as chlamydia, this is a realistic and feasible approach to care, particularly when there is a risk that the young person may not return for follow-up.

Whether providing a mainstream or outreach approach to targeting young men, several factors remain important. Urine samples for diagnosing infection are more popular than urethral swabs. Although more costly with the added disadvantage of not detecting asymptomatic non-specific urethritis, they have the benefit of encouraging more testing for those who are fearful of traditional techniques. In terms of chlamydia control (and, in future, other STIs), urine testing should be the minimal standard offered to sexually active young men. Again, more expensive, single-dose treatments are preferable and these can be administered under observation whilst in the clinic. Single-dose treatments are particularly useful where there are concerns about medication adherence. Getting as many contact details from service users is also important. Essential is a mobile phone number, which most young people generally have. It is preferable to get more than one contact number, as some young people change phones, networks and numbers on a regular basis. Finally, making access to results easier needs to be well thought-out. Novel initiatives include texting or emailing results. Letter results are often inappropriate, as these risk breaking the young person's confidentiality, especially those who still live with parents or carers. Where possible, a range of flexible options should be offered, as it is these small details that can make for a more accessible service, which in turn will increase service reputation and uptake.

Box 8.3: Specific sources of information for boys and young men

- Sexwise helpline offers free, confidential advice on sex, relationships and contraception for under-18s: http://www.ruthinking.co.uk. Tel: 0800 28 29 30
- fpa provides details of sexual health services anywhere in the UK: http://www.fpa.org.uk. Tel: 0845 310 1334
- AVERT is an international HIV and AIDS charity based in the UK that has a Teens section, which includes issues about puberty, sexuality, sex and the Internet, sex and the law, relationships, STIs, HIV and contraception: http://www.avert.org

---

Men who have sex with men

MSM continue to remain a priority for developing culturally appropriate sexual health interventions. Of newly diagnosed STIs among men, MSM accounted for 56% of HIV infections, 22% of gonorrhoea diagnoses and 56% of syphilis diagnoses in 2003.[33] The sustained levels of STI and HIV transmission in MSM are likely to be a result of changing sexual behaviours, particularly the increased proportion reporting unprotected anal intercourse, which has increased significantly each year from 30% in 1996 to 42% in 2000 ($P<0.001$).[37] Another reason for the high level of STIs in the MSM population is that partner notification tends to be less effective in MSM than in heterosexual men, largely reflecting the increased numbers of anonymous sexual contacts that MSM have.[38] Of MSM who do acquire an acute STI, more than 1 in 5 will contract another STI within 12 months.[39]

MSM with frequent partner changes should therefore be actively encouraged to access regular STI screening. In order to facilitate this, many services over the past decade or so have developed targeted MSM-only clinical sessions. This is particularly important in instances where issues of sexuality and associated stigma may be a restricting factor for access. Providing 'gay friendly' or MSM-only services can ensure that MSM service users are not going to be targeted with homophobic attitudes and behaviours from non-MSM service users. MSM clinics can engender a sense of openness so that men are able to freely discuss their concerns without due embarrassment or shame.

Creating a focus on MSM service provision often generates a need for better learning and development opportunities for staff. Providing specific training can result in staff feeling more relaxed and competent to address specific issues such as 'barebacking' (unprotected anal intercourse) and recreational drug use-associated risk behaviours. Health professionals need to be sensitive and adaptive with their prevention messages. Simply telling a gay man to use condoms is not enough. Professionals should be able to have open discussions about what has been coined 'negotiated safety'. This is an agreement between two people in a relationship who want to go through the process of getting ready to stop using condoms. The theory is that both know each other's HIV status and that there is to be no unprotected sex outside the relationship. Some professionals have a cynical view to this approach as it relies on honesty and trust in a relationship. However, individuals need to be supported to make informed decisions; otherwise they are likely to make the decision anyway, possibly without full consideration of the implications.

Health professionals also need to have a good idea about the context of MSM sex and relationships. Amongst other things, they need to have an understanding about recreational drug and alcohol use, peer norms and pressures, HIV serodiscordant relationships, differing sexual practices, and safer-sex negotiation in relationships or one-off anonymous encounters in public sex environments (PSEs). PSEs can include sex on club premises, outdoors in parks (cruising areas) and in public conveniences (cottages). Professionals also need to keep up to date with changing trends in sexual practices and sex-seeking behaviours. The introduction of Internet chat rooms is a good example in which health-promotion specialists have had to redirect resources and ideas about targeting information. Finally, professionals need to know about local points of referral for the voluntary and community sector. These 'third sector' organisations play an essential role in supporting the broader sexual health needs of MSM beyond STI screening and treatment.

Box 8.4: Specific services and sources of information for MSM

- GMFA has a primary objective of preventing HIV infection in gay men through various projects, including the implementation of sexual health-promotion campaigns aimed at black gay men: http://www.metromate.org.uk
- CHAPS is a partnership of community-based organisations, co-ordinated by the Terrence Higgins Trust, carrying out HIV health promotion with gay men in England and Wales: http://www.chapsonline.org.uk
- The NAZ Project supports gay and bisexual men from the Middle East, South Aisia, North Africa, Horn of Africa and Latin America: http://www.naz.org.uk
- Pace is an organisation which responds to the emotional, mental and physical health needs of lesbians and gay men in the greater London area, including counselling related to sex, sexuality and sexual health: http://www.pacehealth.org.uk

Black and minority ethnic men

The UK's black and minority ethnic (BME) populations continue to be disproportionately affected by poor sexual health.[33] The groups affected and their experiences of HIV and STIs vary greatly. Much of the evidence has arisen from studies based on data from GUM clinics and, more recently, HIV and STI surveillance. Findings seem consistent across settings and over time, with generally higher rates of bacterial STIs being reported in black ethnic groups,[40–42] and lower rates in Asian groups than in white groups.[43,44] What has been determined is that individual sexual behaviour is a key determinant of STI transmission risk, but alone does not explain the varying risk across ethnic groups.[45] It may be that race and ethnicity are markers associated with fundamental determinants of health, such as poverty and seeking health care,[46] or that a person's cultural background has a strong influence on his or her sexual attitudes and behaviours,[47] sexual mixing patterns and choices of partner.[48] What is clear is that there are ethnic variations relating to the acquisition and transmission of STIs that warrant specific attention, with a need for targeted and culturally competent prevention interventions.[49] Chief among these approaches are improving STI surveillance and research tools; creating collaborative partnerships with communities; targeting high-risk groups and networks; and improving access to, and the utilisation of, proven effective interventions.[50]

As with STI interventions, there is also a need to develop culturally appropriate responses for the prevention of HIV transmission and acquisition amongst heterosexual minority ethnic groups. Considerable work has already been concentrated on black African groups. However, other groups also require attention, such as South Asians.[51]

Box 8.5: Ten practical tips for sexual health promotion with BME groups[52]

- Have publicity and information materials in any relevant community languages
- Ensure that effective interpretation services are available
- Proactively seek out positive images of people from BME communities
- Do not cover up rates of sexual health problems, in particular BME communities
- Develop and informed understanding of the cultural differences between different BME groups
- Have a diverse range of condoms available
- Place sexual services within a broader health context
- Raise issues of female genital mutilation
- Address local HIV services and HIV-prevention initiatives to support the needs of people from sub-Saharan African countries
- Make strong links with other local BME groups

In terms of MSM from BME groups, of all new diagnoses of HIV in MSM between 1997 and 2002, 12% were in BME MSM.[53] More than half of these probably acquired their infection in the UK, and there is evidence that there is an elevated undiagnosed HIV prevalence in Caribbean-born MSM, highlighting a need for black Caribbean MSM to be prioritised when planning health-promotion initiatives. MSM from BME populations can also experience higher levels of racial and sexual discrimination, with racism coming from the gay community and homophobia coming from the black community. This can lead to isolation from both communities. BME MSM are more likely to report higher sexual risk-taking than other MSM, possibly as a result of the lack of culturally appropriate information, safe spaces and social networks to meet their sexual health needs.

HIV-positive men

There is a strong argument for developing STI care pathways for HIV-positive men. This is because of the increase in sexual risk-taking behaviours and higher STI rates diagnosed in HIV-positive individuals living in the UK. These changes have been most notably seen in HIV-positive MSM.[54–57]

However, sexual health for HIV-positive men is more than just STI screening. Issues related to HIV disclosure, risk reduction in serodiscordant relationships and hepatitis co-infection are amongst the issues unique to those with HIV.[58] An increased rate of sexual problems is also seen in HIV-positive men, warranting more specific sexual health services for this population.[59–61] Although an intervention currently unsupported by empirical research, targeted screening for anal intraepithelial neoplasia (AIN) may be another issue for consideration in the future.[62,63] In addition, the contentious topics of HIV super-infection and sexual transmission of drug-resistant strains of HIV provide further support for informed discussions by specialist HIV sexual health providers.

The question is how best to provide these services. Miles[58] suggests that one means would be to provide a designated, specialist sexual health provider within the HIV setting. However, this can lead to sexual health being compartmentalised away from other aspects of HIV health and social care, as well as de-skilling other

---

Box 8.6: Specific services and sources of information for HIV-positive men

- The Terrence Higgins Trust was one of the first charities to be set up in response to the HIV epidemic and has been providing support services for those affected by HIV ever since: http://www.tht.org.uk
- AIDSMAP is the principal information provider on AIDS and HIV in the UK: http://www.aidsmap.com
- GMFA provide information about sex and being HIV positive: http://www.metromate.org.uk

staff. A more holistic approach would be to integrate the concept of sexual health into the routine elements of HIV care. This would involve all HIV care providers being skilled in conducting routine sexual and reproductive health assessments, providing basic intervention, including engaging clients in HIV/STI-prevention discussions, and/or making onward referral. By introducing and normalising sexual health at all levels of the HIV care trajectory, individuals should feel more comfortable in coming forward with their issues and concerns.

Male sex workers

Male sex work has changed over recent years, with a new growth in the sexual market such as the introduction of Internet chat-rooms, contact magazines and Internet sites advertising 'escort' or 'massage' services. As a result, in some areas, traditional street work has declined, leading to closure of services targeted at this population.[64] Changes in traditional male sex-worker scenes does not mean that male sex work has decreased: quite the opposite – male sex work appears to be a successful occupation for many men, particularly in densely populated urban areas such as London. However, the proportion of men who have ever paid for sex with men remains disproportionate to that of men paying women for sex (0.19% compared with 8.8% of British men surveyed in 2000).[65,66] This is of course a reflection on the proportion of men ever having had sex with another man (5.4% of British men surveyed in 2000).[67]

Although over time there has been little change in sexual risk behaviour in men who sell sex, there is a continued high prevalence of STIs reported in this population.[68] However, it is likely the increased risk of HIV and STIs occurs during non-paying sexual encounters – i.e. more consistent condom use has been reported for anal intercourse with paying partners than non-paying.[69] This has also been the case for female sex workers.[70]

Health professionals should always consider that making active choices to sell sex is not always the situation. There are circumstances where young males are coerced into selling sex or exchanging sex for shelter, drugs or even company. Some of these men have related behavioural and mental health problems, such as drug- and alcohol-dependence issues, law-offending behaviour and self-harm behaviours. As a result, low self-esteem can lead to increased sexual risk behaviours.

Service providers therefore need to cater according to the specific needs of the varying types of sex worker populations. Where there are concentrated populations of 'organised' or 'residential-based' male sex workers, targeted services can facilitate access to regular screening, the provision of condoms and specific advice and support related to sex work. Many of these men may also identify as gay men, and therefore access gay men's sexual health services or services known to be 'gay friendly'.

Where there are street sex-worker scenes, 'outreach' approaches have been successful, particularly joint working partnerships between mainstream sexual health services and community-based health promotion and prevention initiatives. In addition to providing STI/HIV-prevention interventions, community initiatives have been successful in co-ordinating elements of primary health and social care.

Beyond this, generic sexual health services need to provide a confidential, non-judgemental approach to care so that service users are able to disclose their behaviour in relation to both paying and non-paying sexual encounters.

Box 8.7: Specific services and sources of information for male sex workers

- SW5 works with male and transgender sex workers in south west London: http://www.sw5.info
- The Working Men Project provides free, friendly and confidential specialist sexual health services for men who sell sex or work in the commercial male sex industry: http://www.wmplondon.org.uk
- Barnardo's Young Men's Project provides support and advocacy for young males being sexually exploited: http://www.services.barnardos.org.uk/youngmenslondon

---

Male sexual assault and rape

Male rape in Britain did not exist as an offence until the legal definition was changed in 1994. Reported male rape subsequently increased from 150 cases in 1995 to 893 in 2003–2004.[71] The introduction of the Sexual Offences Act (2003) in May 2004 resulted in substantial changes to sexual offences reporting, with new definitions of rape, assault by penetration, sexual assault and causing a person to engage in sexual activity without consent.[72] This means that figures for 2004–2005 are not comparable with those for previous years. Nonetheless, in 2004–2005 there were 1,135 recorded cases of male rape and 2,517 reports of sexual assaults on males, both figures including male children. Of all reported rape, only 8% were accounted to males.[71]

The Home Office has conducted research into the extent and nature of rape and sexual assault of women.[73] The data originated from computerised, self-completion questionnaires included in the 1998 and 2000 British Crime Surveys. These questions were designed to provide the most accurate-ever estimates of the extent and nature of sexual victimisation in England and Wales. The questions were asked of both men and women aged 16–59, but, unfortunately, findings were only ever published from the female respondents.

Although the true prevalence of sexual assault of men in the wider community is not known, one study in a general practice sample reported a 5% lifetime prevalence, with 3% in adulthood.[74] The same study found that non-consensual sexual experiences were associated with a greater prevalence of psychological and alcohol problems, and self-harm. Other studies have shown that men attending

GUM services tend to have experienced a higher prevalence of sexual assault (18% as adults),[75] and men who have sex with men report even higher rates (27.6%).[76]

GUM services have generally been the main clinical point of contact for providing STI screening and psychological support for men who have been sexually assaulted and/or raped, and most see such cases as a priority.[77] However, more specific clinical and forensic services for men have only existed in recent years. This is partly due to the low demand for such services, which itself is likely to have been fuelled by the lack of acknowledgement of male rape, by both the legal system and society in general. Such services include the newly defined sexual assault referral centres (SARCs). SARCs are a one-stop location where victims of sexual assault can receive medical care and counselling while at the same time having the opportunity to assist police investigations, including facilities for a high standard of forensic examination. At present there are only 13 SARCs across England and Wales, although there is a strong commitment to strengthen and extend the SARC network. Over time it is expected that the number of men presenting post-sexual assault to SARCs will increase, but despite significant risk, many may never engage with medical care.[78] This carries an unknown risk of onward HIV and other STI transmission.

Box 8.8: Specific services and sources of information for men who have been sexually assaulted and/or raped

- Survivors UK provides a telephone help-line service offering help and support to adult male victims of sexual abuse and rape. The helpline is also there for the families, partners and friends of men who have experienced sexual abuse and/or rape. Survivors UK also provides face-to-face counselling, a support group in London, a range of recommended reading for survivors, partners and family of survivors and health and social care professionals, and a range of useful weblinks: http://www.survivorsuk.org.uk
- Operation Emotion was set up by the survivors of one of Britain's most prolific paedophiles, to provide one-to-one counselling, group support and counselling, family support and counselling, and email support: http://www.operationemotion.co.uk
- The National Association of Male Sexual Assault Services (NAMSAS) is a collective of agencies that offer a service to men who have suffered sexual assault/abuse at any time in their lives. NAMSAS aims to address the issues men face and work on collaborative projects to provide appropriate services for them : http://www.namsas.org.uk
- The National Association for People Abused in Childhood provides support through the provision of materials and the listing of local groups for adults who were abused as children: http://www.napac.org.uk

FUTURE SEXUAL HEALTH SERVICE PROVISION FOR MEN

Sexual health has finally reached priority on the public health policy agenda, but pressure needs to remain constant in order to maintain an awareness about the specific issues relating to men's sexual health. There is an ongoing requirement to explore the sexual health needs of men so that innovative approaches to addressing these needs can be developed. In particular, the following issues are raised:

- There is a need for better information about the range of sexual health services available to men, with male-targeted media playing a bigger role.
- There is a need to develop and use more non-invasive STI screening approaches that can improve the user experience and promote service uptake by those reluctant to undergo traditional screening methods.
- There is a need to identify and use culturally appropriate community STI/HIV screening venues for men. As previously mentioned, the majority of screening sites in the national chlamydia screening programme are centred on women. There is an urgent need to offer screening to men where they study, work and socialise. Any intervention should also take into account the wide variance in community norms, particularly in relation to black and minority ethnic groups and those from different religious or spiritual backgrounds. There is a need to work with minority communities to develop socially appropriate responses to local sexual health problems.
- There is a need to explore more interventions that enable rapid treatment, such as 'partner interventions', where individuals who are known to have an STI are given treatment to give to their partners.
- Current contraception choices continue to restrict the responsibility of men in the prevention of unintended pregnancies. There is an urgent need for new, safe and reliable methods of contraception to be developed for men. This includes the development of hormonal and other pharmacological agents.
- There is a need to develop better care pathways for men with sexual dysfunction. At present a man can be assessed by a GUM practitioner, but may need to be referred to someone else to receive ongoing treatment. Men need to have clearer information about what their options are and who can provide them.
- Men with physical and sensory disabilities, learning difficulties and mental health problems need to have their sexual health needs addressed.
- There is an urgent need to address the sexual health needs of men within prisons and youth-offending institutes. Studies have identified chlamydia in up to 13% of the male prison population.[79] Successful, nurse-led sexual health services have been developed within prison services in partnership with local GUM clinics. Further models should be developed and rolled out.

All of these interventions (and more) are feasible, but the main restriction for better services for men centres on funding. Mainstream NHS sexual health services are currently facing significant financial challenges. Services are being placed under increased pressure to contain, and in some instances, reduce costs. This is set against a backdrop of an increasing demand for services, increasing costs of technology and treatments, new unaccounted cost pressures such as post-exposure prophylaxis, pressure to meet policy targets and human resource issues such as recruitment and retention difficulties, and decreasing learning and development budgets. As a result, services are having to make difficult decisions that can lead to a reduction in 'non-essential' services. For example, the use of clinical psychology services within some GUM clinics are moving towards having strict criteria for accepting referrals. Priorities lie with those who are at most risk of self or public harm that is directly related to STIs, HIV and other blood-borne infections, leaving those with less critical public health consequences, such as sexual dysfunction, on long waiting lists or being referred towards independent or community-based organisations. Such issues are of course counterproductive to the all-embracing definition of sexual healthcare.

As a result, there is likely to be an increased emphasis on developing partnerships and clear referral pathways between NHS and non-NHS providers. This is likely to happen as a result of necessity rather than choice, particularly in relation to the recent proposals for changing the role of the public sector from being less of a direct provider to being more of a commissioner of services.[80,81] This issue is largely contentious, with the current focus of debate being around the use of the commercial sector, with controversy over 'privatising NHS staff'. Nonetheless, this process has already begun in sexual health, with a high-street commercial pharmacy (Boots) recently being commissioned by the NHS to provide chlamydia screening and treatment over the counter.[82] The advantage of using independent sector providers such as Boots is that they are already in position on the high street to provide NHS-quality chlamydia testing. This means costs to the taxpayer are kept down and there is no need to draw on staff from other areas of the NHS.

However, there is little being said about the use of voluntary and community organisations (VCOs), or the 'third sector' as it has been called. These organisations already play a pivotal role in the sexual health arena, particularly for targeted groups of the population such as HIV-positive people and adolescents. For example, the Terrence Higgins Trust have extensive experience in engaging volunteers to provide HIV home care, advice, information and counselling services, and Brook Advisory Centres have 40 years' experience of providing professional sexual and reproductive health advice through specially trained doctors, nurses, counsellors, and outreach and information workers, to over 100,000 young people each year.

The key to better integration with existing NHS services will probably rest with getting future commissioning arrangements correct. If commissioning arrangements are not right, there is a risk that competition for funding could invariably result in tensions between those services who should be working together, as well as a range of concerns over quality and profiteering.

In summary, for services to adequately cater for men, there is a need for continued political awareness and commitment, increased empowerment and involvement of male service users in services decisions, and a range of innovative, culturally appropriate and co-ordinated approaches that are commissioned with clearly defined care pathways between the various public, independent, voluntary and community sector providers.

REFERENCES

1 Social Exclusion Unit. *Teenage pregnancy.* London: The Stationery Office; 1999.
2 Department of Health. *The national strategy for sexual health and HIV.* London: Department of Health; 2001.
3 Department of Health. *The national strategy for sexual health and HIV: implementation action plan.* London: Department of Health; 2002.
4 Department of Health. *Effective commissioning of sexual health and HIV services: a sexual health and HIV commissioning toolkit for primary care trusts and local authorities.* London: Department of Health; 2003.
5 MedFASH. *Recommended standards for sexual health services.* London: Medical Foundation for AIDS & Sexual Health; 2005.
6 Department of Health. *National service framework for children, young people and maternity services.* London: Department of Health; 2004.
7 Department for Education and Skills. *Every child matters: change for children.* London: DfES; 2004.
8 Department of Health. *Choosing health: making healthy choices easier.* London: Department of Health; 2004.
9 Darroch J, Myers L and Cassell J. Sex differences in the experience of testing positive for genital chlamydia infection: a qualitative study with implications for public health and for a national screening programme. *Sex Transm Infect* 2003; **79**(5): 372–373.
10 Cassell J, Mercer CH, Sutcliffe L, Brook G, Jungman E, Ross G, *et al. Sexual behaviour and risk of ongoing transmission in symptomatic patients attending genitourinary medicine clinics* (Oral presentation O12a). 11th Annual Conference of the British HIV Association with the British Association for Sexual Health and HIV, Dublin, Ireland; 2005.
11 Sutcliffe L, Brook G, Mensah J and Cassell J. Why does it take men so long to get to clinic? A qualitative study of heterosexual men attending an urban sexual health clinic (Poster presentation P126). BASHH/ASTDA Spring Meeting, Bath. *Int J STD AIDS* 2004; **15**(Suppl 1): 40–41.
12 Health Protection Agency. Update on the roll-out of the National Chlamydia Screening Programme (NCSP). *CDR Weekly* 2005; **15**(26): 7–9.
13 World Health Organization (WHO). International WHO technical consultation on sexual health (28–31 January 2002). [Internet] Available from: http://www.who.int/reproductive-health [accessed 2002].

14 Royal College of Nursing. *Sexuality and sexual health in nursing practice*. London: RCN; 2000.

15 Johnson AM, Mercer CH, Erens B, Copas AJ, McManus S, Wellings K, *et al*. Sexual behaviour in Britain: partnerships, practices, and HIV risk behaviours. *Lancet* 2001; **358**(9296): 1835–1842.

16 Mercer CH, Fenton KA, Johnson AM, Wellings K, Macdowall W, McManus S, *et al*. Sexual function problems and help seeking behaviour in Britain: national probability sample survey. *BMJ* 2003; **327**(7412): 426–427.

17 Royal Commission on Venereal Diseases. Final report of the Commissioners (Cmnd 8189). London: HMSO; 1916.

18 Health Protection Agency. All new episodes seen at GUM clinics: 1999–2003. Country specific tables. [Internet] http://www.hpa.org.uk [accessed 04/11/05].

19 Department of Health. *NHS Trusts and Primary Care Trusts (sexually transmitted diseases) directions 2000*. London: Department of Health; 2000.

20 Miles K, Penny N, Mercey DE and Power R. A postal survey to identify and describe nurse-led clinics in Genitourinary Medicine services across England. *Sex Transm Infect* 2002; **78**(2): 98–100.

21 Handy P. Nurse-directed services in genitourinary medicine. *Nurs Stand* 2002; **17**(11): 33–38.

22 Harindra V, Tobin JM and Tucker LJ. Triage clinics: a way forward in genitourinary medicine. *Int J STD AIDS* 2001; **12**: 295–298.

23 Miles K, Penny N, Mercey DE and Power R. Sexual health clinics for women led by specialist nurses or senior house officers in a central London GUM service: a randomised controlled trial. *Sex Transm Infect* 2002; **78**(2): 93–97.

24 Miles K, Penny N, Power R and Mercey D. Comparing doctor- and nurse-led care in a sexual health clinic: patient satisfaction questionnaire. *J Adv Nurs* 2003; **42**(1): 64–72.

25 Martin D, Barter J and Pittrof R. *Experience with the test not talk (TNT) clinic for asymptomatic men* (Poster presentation P3). 11th Annual Conference of the British HIV Association with the British Association for Sexual Health and HIV, Dublin, Ireland, 2005.

26 McQuillan O, Hewart R and Morgan E. *Mobile phone text messaging to give results to patients in a district general hospital genitourinary medicine clinic* (Poster presentation P14). 11th Annual Conference of the British HIV Association with the British Association for Sexual Health and HIV, Dublin, Ireland, 2005.

27 Clarke J, Taylor Y and Harkin P. *Results by text – preferred by patients, transforming work patterns* (Poster presentation P13). 11th Annual Conference of the British HIV Association with the British Association for Sexual Health and HIV, Dublin, Ireland, 2005.

28 Menon-Johansson A, Mcnaught F, Mandalia S and Sullivan A. *Test > text > treatment: text messaging service (TMS) improves the time to treatment of* Chlamydia trachomatis *infection and reduces the cost of result provision* (Poster presentation P81a). 11th Annual Conference of the British HIV Association with the British Association for Sexual Health and HIV, Dublin, Ireland, 2005.

29 Department of Health. *NHS Contraceptive Services, England: 2001–2002*. London: Department of Health; 2002.

30 Pearson S. Men's use of sexual health services. *J Fam Plann Reprod Health Care* 2003; **29**(4): 190–194.

31 Teenage Pregnancy Unit. *Guidance for developing contraception and sexual health advice services to reach boys and young men.* London: Department of Health; 2000.

32 Walton M and Anderson RA. Hormonal contraception in men. *Curr Drug Targets Immune Endocr Metabol Disord* 2005; **5**(3): 249–257.

33 The UK Collaborative Group for HIV and STI Surveillance. *Focus on prevention. HIV and other sexually transmitted infections in the United Kingdom in 2003.* London: Health Protection Agency Centre for Infections; 2004.

34 Pearson S. Promoting sexual health services to young men: findings from focus group discussions. *J Fam Plann Reprod Health Care* 2003; **29**(4): 194–198.

35 Centre for HIV & Sexual Health Services. Undercover – Young People's Sexual Health Service Evaluation Scheme. Sheffield. [Internet] http://www.sexualhealthsheffield.co.uk/projects.html [accessed 04/11/05].

36 Department of Health. *Best practice guidance for doctors and other health professionals on the provision of advice and treatment to young people under 16 on contraception, sexual and reproductive health.* London: DoH; 2004.

37 Dodds JP, Mercey DE, Parry JV and Johnson AM. Increasing risk behaviour and high levels of undiagnosed HIV infection in a community sample of homosexual men. *Sex Transm Infect* 2004; **80**(3): 236–240.

38 Coleman C, Bergin C, Hopkins S and Mulchay F. The effectiveness of partner notification for gonococcal infection: a comparison between men who have sex with men and heterosexual men (Poster presentation P78). BASHH/ASTDA Spring Meeting, Bath. *Int J STD AIDS* 2004; **15**(Suppl 1): 28.

39 Hughes G, Brady AR, Catchpole MA, Fenton KA, Rogers PA, Kinghorn GR, *et al.* Characteristics of those who repeatedly acquire sexually transmitted infections: a retrospective cohort study of attendees at three urban sexually transmitted disease clinics in England. *Sex Transm Dis* 2001; **28**(7): 379–386.

40 Low N, Daker-White G, Barlow D and Pozniak AL. Gonorrhoea in inner London: results of a cross sectional study. *BMJ* 1997; **314**(7096): 1719–1723.

41 Lacey CJ, Merrick DW, Bensley DC and Fairley I. Analysis of the sociodemography of gonorrhoea in Leeds, 1989–1993. *BMJ* 1997; **314**(7096): 1715–1718.

42 Low N, Sterne JA and Barlow D. Inequalities in rates of gonorrhoea and chlamydia between black ethnic groups in south east London: cross sectional study. *Sex Transm Infect* 2001; **77**(1): 15–20.

43 Hughes G, Brady AR, Catchpole MA, Fenton KA, Rogers PA, Kinghorn GR, *et al.* Characteristics of those who repeatedly acquire sexually transmitted infections: a retrospective cohort study of attendees at three urban sexually transmitted disease clinics in England. *Sex Transm Dis* 2001; **28**(7): 379–386.

44 Cliffe S, Mortimer J, McGarrigle C, Boisson E, Parry JV, Turner A, *et al.* Surveillance for the impact in the UK of HIV epidemics in South Asia. *Ethn Health* 1999; **4**(1, 2): 5–18.

45 Fenton KA, Mercer CH, McManus S, Erens B, Wellings K, Macdowall W, *et al.* Ethnic variations in sexual behaviour in Great Britain and risk of sexually transmitted infections: a probability survey. *Lancet* 2005; **365**(9466): 1246–1255.

46 Freeman HP. Poverty, race, racism and survival. *AIDS Educ Prev* 1993; **3**: 145–149.

47 Cleland J and Ferry B. *Sexual behaviour and AIDS in the developing world.* London: Taylor and Francis; 1995.

48 Fenton K, Johnson AM and Nicoll A. Race, ethnicity, and sexual health. *BMJ* 1997; **314**(7096): 1703–1704.

49 Fenton KA, Mercer CH, McManus S, Erens B, Wellings K, Macdowall W, *et al.* Ethnic variations in sexual behaviour in Great Britain and risk of sexually transmitted infections: a probability survey. *Lancet* 2005; **365**(9466): 1246–1255.

50 Fenton KA. Strategies for improving sexual health in ethnic minorities. *Curr Opin Infect Dis* 2001; **14**(1): 63–69.

51 Sethi G, Lacey CJ, Fenton KA, Williams IG, Fox E, Sabin CA, *et al.* South Asians with HIV in London: Is it time to rethink sexual health service delivery to meet the needs of heterosexual ethnic minorities? *Sex Transm Infect* 2004; **80**(1): 75–76.

52 Department of Health. *Fact Sheet Nine – 10 Practical tips for sexual health promotion with black and minority ethnic groups. Effective sexual health promotion: a toolkit for Primary Care Trusts and others working in the field of promoting good sexual health and HIV prevention.* London: Department of Health; 2003.

53 Dougan S, Elford J, Brown AE, Sinka K, Evans BG, Gill ON, *et al.* Epidemiology of HIV among black and minority ethnic men who have sex with men in England and Wales. *Sex Transm Infect* 2005; **81**(4): 345–350.

54 Ivens D and Patel M. Incidence and presentation of early syphilis diagnosed in HIV-positive gay men attending a central London outpatients' department. *Int J STD AIDS* 2005; **16**(3): 201–202.

55 Dodds JP, Mercey DE, Parry JV and Johnson AM. Increasing risk behaviour and high levels of undiagnosed HIV infection in a community sample of homosexual men. *Sex Transm Infect* 2004; **80**(3): 236–240.

56 Hutchinson J, Estcourt C, Imrie J and Fenton KA. The sexual health needs of HIV-positive people. *Int J STD AIDS* 2003; **14**(7): 500–501.

57 Fenton KA. Sexual health and HIV positive individuals: emerging lessons from the recent outbreaks of infectious syphilis in England. *Commun Dis Public Health* 2002; **5**(1): 4–6.

58 Miles K. Sexual health in the HIV setting (Editorial). *HIV Nurs* 2004; **4**(3): 1.

59 Cove J and Petrak J. Factors associated with sexual problems in HIV-positive gay men. *Int J STD AIDS* 2004; **15**(11): 732–736.

60 Goldmeier D and Lamba H. Sexual dysfunction in HIV-positive individuals. *Int J STD AIDS* 2003; **14**(1): 63–64.

61 Lamba H, Goldmeier D, Mackie NE and Scullard G. Antiretroviral therapy is associated with sexual dysfunction and with increased serum oestradiol levels in men. *Int J STD AIDS* 2004; **15**(4): 234–237.

62 Klencke BJ and Palefsky JM. Anal cancer: an HIV-associated cancer. *Hematol Oncol Clin North Am* 2003; **17**(3): 859–872.

63 Martin F and Bower M. Anal intraepithelial neoplasia in HIV positive people. *Sex Transm Infect* 2001; **77**(5): 327–331.

64 Castro-Sanchez E, Tyner C, LeBray A, Miles K and Mercey D. Outreach services for male sex workers: do we still need them? (Poster presentation P108). BASHH/ASTDA Spring Meeting, Bath. *Int J STD AIDS* 2004; **15**(Suppl 1): 36.

65 Ward H. Who pays for sex? An analysis of the increasing prevalence of female commercial sex contacts among men in Britain. *Sex Transm Infect* 2005; **81**: 467–471.

66 Mercer CH. Estimates from NATSAL survey on percentage of men reporting to have ever paid another man for sex (Personal Communication, 2005).

67 Johnson AM, Mercer CH, Erens B, Copas AJ, McManus S, Wellings K, *et al*. Sexual behaviour in Britain: partnerships, practices, and HIV risk behaviours. *Lancet* 2001; **358**(9296): 1835–1842.

68 Sethi G, Holden B, Gaffney J, Greene L and Ward H. HIV, sexually transmitted infections and risk behaviours in male sex workers in London over a 10-year period (Oral presentation O21). BASHH/ASTDA Spring Meeting, Bath. *Int J STD AIDS* 2004; **15**(Suppl 1): 6.

69 Ziersch A, Gaffney J and Tomlinson DR. STI prevention and the male sex industry in London: evaluating a pilot peer education programme. *Sex Transm Infect* 2000; **76**(6): 447–453.

70 Ward H, Day S, Mezzone J, Dunlop L, Donegan C, Farrar S, *et al*. Prostitution and risk of HIV: female prostitutes in London. *BMJ* 1993; **307**(6900): 356–358.

71 Home Office. *The British crime survey.* London: Home Office Publications; 2005.

72 Home Office. *Sexual Offences Act 2003.* London: The Stationery Office; 2003.

73 Myhill A and Allen J. *Rape and sexual assault of women: the extent and nature of the problem.* Home Office Research Study 237. London: Home Office; 2002.

74 Coxell A, King M, Mezey G and Gordon D. Lifetime prevalence, characteristics, and associated problems of non-consensual sex in men: cross sectional survey. *BMJ* 1999; **318**(7187): 846–850.

75 Coxell AW, King MB, Mezey GC and Kell P. Sexual molestation of men: interviews with 224 men attending a genitourinary medicine service. *Int J STD AIDS* 2000; **11**(9): 574–578.

76 Hickson FC, Davies PM, Hunt AJ, Weatherburn P, McManus TJ and Coxon AP. Gay men as victims of nonconsensual sex. *Arch Sex Behav* 1994; **23**(3): 281–294.

77 Obeyesekera S, Jones K, Forster G, Welch J, Brook G and Daniels D. Management of rape/sexual assault cases within genitourinary medicine clinics (Poster presentation P105). BASHH/ASTDA Spring Meeting, Bath. *Int J STD AIDS* 2004; **15**(Suppl 1): 35.

78 Reeves I, Jawad R and Welch J. Risk of undiagnosed infection in men attending a sexual assault referral centre. *Sex Transm Infect* 2004; **80**(6): 524–525.

79 Winston A, Matthews G, Portsmouth S, Mandalia S and Daniels D. Chlamydia prevalence in male prisoners at a young offenders institute. *Sex Transm Infect* 2003; **79**(Suppl 1): A15.

80 Department of Health. *Commissioning a patient-led NHS.* London: Department of Health; 2005.

81 Department of Health. *Creating a patient-led NHS – delivering the NHS improvement plan.* London: Department of Health; 2005.

82 Department of Health. *Boots selected to provide free chlamydia screening for 16–24 year olds across the capital.* Press Release 2005/0294. London: Department of Health; 2005.

83 Hancock J. Can mainstream services learn from male only sexual health pilot projects? *Sex Transm Infect* 2004; **80**(6): 484–487.

Index

adolescence 19, 85, 88–9, 123–6
age 8, 46, 76–7
    and erectile dysfunction (ED) 59–60, 67
    and premature ejaculation (PE) 71
    and syphilis 49
Africans 95–101, 106, 112, 127–8
Afro-Caribbeans *see* Caribbeans
age of consent 47
AIDS *see* HIV
alcohol 21, 22, 32, 66, 89
allergies 50–1
Alzheimer's disease 67
antibiotics 50, 52, 125
antidepressants 66, 72–3
anxiety 63, 65, 69, 71–6, 84, 118
arthritis 47, 67
Asians 94–7, 101, 107–12, 128
atherosclerosis 64–5
azithromycin 48

Bangladeshis 95, 110
bisexuality 30, 84, 127
black and minority ethnic (BME) *see* ethnicity
body image 63, 74, 77
British Association for Sexual Health and HIV 46–7

cancer, general 9, 15, 21–3, 65
    in males, underpublicized 22
car accidents 19

cardiovascular disease 18, 64
Caribbeans 7, 38, 42, 94–102, 129
    and STIs 49, 97–107
Centre for Disease Surveillance and Control (CDSC) 50
charities 9
check-ups 15
chemotherapy 44–5
chlamydia 47–9
    and ethnicity 97
    presentation 47–8
    prevalence 47
    testing for 47–8, 116
    treating 48
    in young men 46, 123
Choosing Health: Making Healthy Choices Easier 116
class 17, 64, 84
condoms 9, 52, 71–2, 87–90, 100–6
    and HIV 87–90, 127
    and lifestyle 89
    and prostitution 88–9
    and sexual pleasure 89–90
confidentiality 46–7, 75, 120–6, 131
contraception 48, 52, 85, 117–19, 122–6, 133
culture 19–20, 73, 75

death
    and employment 18
    fear of 5, 86
    life expectancy 18–19, 31, 41, 86, 93
    rates 19–20

definitions *see* sexual health
denial of illness 17–18
Department of Health 15, 22, 40, 48, 124
depression 18, 65
deprivation 8, 14, 20, 24, 42, 64, 84
 and gonorrhoea 49
 and masculinity 17
diabetes mellitus 65, 70, 72, 95
diet 22, 32, 66
doxycycline 48
drug use 32, 66, 74, 89, 126

eating disorders 15–16, 21, 74
education, sexual 5, 31–2, 43–4, 84
and ethnicity 96–106
 future of 9
 negative effects 89
embarrassment 15–16, 59, 75–8
emotions 8, 17
employment 18, 20
endocrine disorders 65
epydidymitis 47
Equality Act (2007) vii
erectile dysfunction (ED) vi–vii, 41, 58
 and age 59–60
 and alcohol 66
 assessment 67–70
 causes 62–7
 consequences 7
 defined 59
 and diabetes mellitus 65
 and endocrine disorders 65
 medication 66
 and penile abnormality 67
 perception 59
 physiology 60–2
 and psychology 62–4
 and renal disease 66–7
 and smoking 65, 66
 and surgery 66–7

and Viagra 29
ethnicity 3, 7–8, 20–1, 128–9, 133
 and cancer 38, 42
 and culture 93–4
 defining 94
 diversity 96
 and education 96–106
 and gonorrhoea 49
 and HIV infection 46, 96, 128–9
 and immigration 98
 and inequality in healthcare 95
 lack of research 96
 and masculinity 17
 racism 20, 94–6, 129
 sensitivity 95–6
 and STIs 46, 128–9
 terminology 94–5
exercise 40, 66
exhibitionism 58

family planning 5, 55
female doctors 20–1
female sexual health 15–16
 domination of 22, 27–8, 116–17
foreplay 71, 77

gender difference
 conditioning 19, 28
 and healthcare 22–3, 46
 and Islam 20
 and sexual repression 28, 84
 stereotyping 13–14, 16–18, 30, 73, 77, 83–5
Gender Equality Duty vii
genetics 31, 38, 64, 95
genital warts 46, 123
 presentation 51–2
 treatment 52
genito-urinary medicine (GUM) clinics 5, 46, 97, 102, 120–1

future 133–5
and gender 31
waiting times 116
gonorrhoea 46, 123
and ethnicity 49, 97
prevalence 48
treatment 49
government policy 14–15
GPs 20–1, 47–9, 52, 118, 122
guilt 3

health groups 31
Health Protection Agency (HPA) 46,
97
healthcare, general 1–9, 22–3, 76, 117
improving 9, 14
heterosexuality 30, 84–5, 116–17
HIV 46–7, 129–30
and cancer 42
care 5, 115
and condoms 87–90
context 47
diagnosing 115
dominates sexual health 27, 38
emergence of vi, 1–2, 3, 89
and ethnicity 96–107
and homosexuality 30
impact of 3–4, 38
improved treatment 46
and male prostitution 130
prevention 30, 115
and race 46
in relationships 90
research into 4–5, 27
holistic sexual healthcare 2, 5–7
difficulties with 6
homosexuality *see* men who have sex
with men (MSM)
hormonal therapy 41
HPVs *see* genital warts
hyperlipidaemia 45, 65

hyperprolactinaemia 65
hypertension 29, 45, 65
hyperthyroidism 65
hypoactive sexual desire disorder
(HSDD) 58, 73–4
hypogonadism 65, 67, 73
hypothyroidism 65

immigration 98
impotence *see* erectile dysfunction (ED)
income 8, 14, 20, 24, 42, 64, 84
and gonorrhoea 49
and masculinity 17
inhibited male orgasm 72–3
insomnia 18
integration 2
intensive therapy 78
International Men's Health Database
31–2
International Men's Health Week
31–2
internet 41–2, 46, 87, 121, 125–7

Klinefelter's syndrome 42

language barriers 20–1
libido *see* sexual desire
life expectancy 18–19, 86
lifestyle 1, 4, 18, 20, 22, 32, 66, 95

Macmillan Cancer Relief 42
male breast cancer 15
marginalisation 3–4, 30, 36, 39
marriage 17–18, 45, 84
masculinity
and age 83
and aggression 17–18
crisis in 16

masculinity – continued
   definitions 83
   and dependence 17–18
   and deprivation 17
   nature of 14
   peer pressure 17
   and psychology 16
   and race 17
   and self-neglect 17–19, 22–3, 32,
      44, 117
   stereotyping 13–14, 16–18, 30, 73,
      77, 83–5
   stigmas 15–16, 73, 76
   study of 15
masturbation 3, 72, 77, 85, 123
men's studies 14–15
men who have sex with men (MSM)
      46–9, 52, 84–5, 116, 126–9
   and AIDS 3, 30, 49, 126
   and gonorrhoea 48, 126
   homophobia 126, 129
   stereotypes 85
   and syphilis 49, 126
multiple sclerosis 65

National Chlamydia Screening
      Programme 47, 117
National Health Service (NHS) 116
   lack of support for men's initiatives
      22, 134
   reform 118
National Service Framework for
      Children, Young People and
      Maternity Services 116
National Sexual Activity and Lifestyle
      study 85
National Strategy for Sexual Health
      and HIV (NSSHH) 7–8, 15, 48,
      115, 118
National Teenage Pregnancy Strategy
      115

NEED (Nurse education in erectile
      dysfunction) 69
neurological disorders 62, 65–6
nocturnal emissions 72

oestrogen 18
orchidectomy 41–2, 45

paedophilia 58, 132
Pakistanis 95–7, 107–8, 110
parents 17, 22, 85, 107–8, 112, 122–6
Parkinson's disease 65
Paroxetine 72
penicillin 50–1
penis size 44, 87
personalisation of sexual healthcare
      2–3, 5
Peyronie's disease 67
pituitary adenomas 73
pleasure, sexual 5, 6, 37–8, 63, 71, 84,
      89–90, 118
PLISSIT 76, 78
poverty *see* deprivation
pregnancy
   teenage 116
   unplanned 2, 6–7, 115–16, 122
premature ejaculation (PE) 69
   and age 71
   defined 70–1
   treatments 71–2
preventative healthcare
   lack of 30–1
privacy 1–3
prolactin 65, 73–4
prostate cancer 9
   incidence 38–9
   natural history 38–9, 41
   presentation 39–40
   screening 39–41
   stages 39

survival rate 38–9
treatment 41–2
Prostate Cancer Charity, The 42
prostate-specific antigen (PSA) testing 38–42
accuracy 40
prostitution 3, 88
male 130–1
psychology 5, 9, 29, 37–8, 73
and erectile dysfunction (ED) 62–4
and masculinity 16
psychosexuality 9, 16, 75–8
and erectile dysfunction (ED) 62
puberty 43, 85, 123, 126

race see ethnicity
racism 20, 94–6, 129
radiotherapy 41, 44, 131–2
rape 74–5, 77, 123, 131–3
rapid ejaculation see premature ejaculation (PE)
rectal infections 49
Reiter's Syndrome 47
relationships 17–18, 45, 58–9, 84
and HIV 90
trust 88–9
religion 7, 20–1, 64, 75, 84, 94–7, 111, 133
renal disease 64, 66–7
research into sexual health
and gender 27–8
growth of 15
impediments to 3, 8
importance 7
shortage of 4–5, 7, 27–30, 86
responsibility 7
reticence 3, 21–2, 32–3, 44, 74, 117
retrograde ejaculation 72
risk taking 9

seeking healthcare 16, 31–2
selective serotonin reuptake inhibitors (SSRIs) 72, 73
self-harm 74
self-neglect 17–19, 22–3, 32, 44, 117
Sertraline 72
sexual abuse 58, 74, 84, 132
sexual addiction 58
sexual assault see rape
sexual behaviour 9, 32
sexual desire 41, 69
levels 73–4
reduced 69
sexual dysfunction
defining 58
prevalence 58–9
sexual health
complexity 8, 58
defining 6–7, 37–8
and general health 9
prevalence 118
Sexual Health Inventory for Men (SHIM) 68–9
sexual health services 120–32
access to 14
cost 7
defining 117–19
fragmented 6
future 133–5
improvement 9
sexual pleasure see pleasure, sexual
sexual politics 15
sexuality 9, 30
sexually transmitted infections (STIs) 2–3
and ethnicity 49, 97
and gender 30–1
incidence 45–7, 115–16
and male prostitution 130
rise in numbers of 5, 32, 46
screening 23, 39–43, 47–50, 117–18, 124–33

STIs – continued
  social consequences 7, 38
  symptoms 45
  treatment 46–7, 115
sildenafil *see* Viagra
single dose treatments 125
smoking 5, 21
  and erectile dysfunction (ED) 65, 66
sociology 3, 7–8, 14
  and change 8
  importance of 16–17
sperm storage 44
spinal cord injury 65
stroke 65
suicide 19
surgery 41, 44, 66–7, 70, 72, 75, 77
surveys 2–3
  limitations 7
syphilis
  presentation 50
  prevalence 49–50
  treatment 50–1

testicular cancer 9, 21–2, 123
  cure rates 43
  following up 45
  incidence 42

  pain 44
  presentation 42–3
  screening 43
  treating 44–5
  types 44
testicular self-examination 21, 43
testosterone 18–19, 65, 70, 73–4
theories of sexual health 6

unemployment 18, 20
unplanned pregnancy *see* pregnancy
unprotected sex 31
urethral discharge 48
urethritis 47, 123, 125
urinary control 41

vascular disease 64
Viagra 29, 59, 70
Victorian era 3, 20
violence 19
virginity 85

waiting times 116
World Health Organization (WHO) 2,
  5, 6, 33, 39